# MASTERING
# BEAUTY

A Rare Glimpse into the Private Lives of
Renowned Cosmetic Doctors Who Share Insights
and Advice on the Complex Quest for Beauty

We exist only to discover
beauty:

all else is a form of waiting.

Khalil Gibran

Published by

benton buckley books
be bold.

www.bentonbuckleybooks.com

Principal Publisher: Beth Buckley
Lead Writer & Managing Editor: Rosalie Wilson
Graphics: Morganne Stewart
Production Manager: Erica Core

FIRST EDITION

Distributed by Independent Publishers Group
800.888.4741

PUBLISHER'S DATA

MASTERING BEAUTY
A Rare Glimpse into the Private Lives of
Renowned Cosmetic Doctors Who Share Insights
and Advice on the Complex Quest for Beauty

Library of Congress Cataloging-in-Publication Data
has been applied for.
ISBN: 978-0-9964721-9-7

For information about custom editions, special sales, or
premium and corporate books, please contact benton
buckley books at bebold@bentonbuckleybooks.com.

First Printing 2018
10 9 8 7 6 5 4 3 2 1

PHOTOGRAPHY CREDITS

*Dr. Ashley Gordon's photography by* David Heisler Photography
*Dr. James Grotting's photography by* Roger Stephenson
*Dr. Clyde Ishii's photography by* Gabe Cabagbag
*Dr. John Koutsoyiannis's photography by* Matthew Sowa Photography
*Dr. Charles Lee's photography by* Leon Tang
*Dr. Sheila Nazarian's photography by* Emily Sandifer
*Dr. Anna Petropoulos's photography by* Cordero Studios, Michael Chu, & Shelkovitz Studios
*Dr. Tracy Pfeifer's photography by* Ken Pao
*Dr. Marta Rendon's photography by* Anthony Humphries & Guy Brooks Photography
*Dr. Adam Rubinstein's photography by* Troy Campbell Studio
*Dr. Robyn Siperstein-Paul's photography by* Troy Campbell Studio
*Dr. Armando Soto's photography by* Stephen Allen Photography
*Dr. Charles Thorne's photography courtesy of* Dr. Charles Thorne
*Dr. Jennifer Walden's photography by* Mary Jane Starke
*Dr. Richard Warren's photography by* Michael O'Shea Photography & Kathryn Langsford

# Mastering Beauty

"Why is it that we say 'beauty is in the eye of the beholder?' Very simply, it is because we innately know beauty when we see it, but we can't exactly define it. It defies specific characterization and transcends gender, culture, age, and time. Wall Street and marketing firms exploit it but they don't create it. We all admire it and seek it. Beauty makes the human condition better. Although it relates to the intrinsic qualities of an object or a person, it evokes a response in the beholder that is visceral, and takes almost no time to imprint itself on the mind and psyche of the person who is taking it all in instantly. It is hard to imagine life without beauty."

Jim Grotting

# MASTERS OF BEAUTY

DR. CHARLES THORNE

DR. ASHLEY GORDON

DR. JAMES GROTTING

DR. CLYDE ISHII

DR. JOHN KOUTSOYIANNIS

DR. CHARLES LEE

DR. SHEILA NAZARIAN

DR. ANNA PETROPOULOS

DR. TRACY PFEIFER

DR. MARTA RENDON

DR. ADAM RUBINSTEIN

DR. ROBYN SIPERSTEIN-PAUL

DR. ARMANDO SOTO

DR. JENNIFER WALDEN

DR. RICHARD WARREN

# DISCUSSION TOPICS

"When you look at something or someone beautiful, you're overcome with peace, you feel good, and your brain relaxes because your eyes are experiencing what your soul craves: harmony."

Marta Rendon

"Beauty doesn't have to
be defined. It simply is."

John Koutsoyiannis

# FOREWORD

P lastic surgery, and the beauty business in general, is a fascinating field. Arbitrarily divided into "reconstructive" surgery and "cosmetic" surgery, plastic surgery is a schizophrenic specialty. While a patient who suffers a severe facial injury from a motor vehicle accident clearly represents a reconstructive situation, and the woman who desires the improvement of aging changes in the face clearly represents a cosmetic situation, what about the child who is born without an ear? Is construction of the ear reconstructive or cosmetic? It's obviously both. And that's what is so interesting about the face. The function of the face is to look like a face, and making any separation between what is reconstructive and what is cosmetic is utterly impossible.

*Mastering Beauty* is an unprecedented collection of profiles on some of the world's foremost doctors of cosmetic surgery, dermatology, and dentistry. Readers learn about the personal and professional lives of the experts. The book explores the various philosophies of beauty and presents advice on important topics. No field has more "fake news" than the beauty business, so how does the consumer sort out what is real and what is poppycock? The

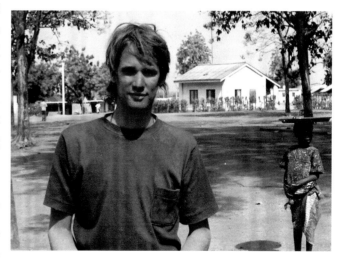

beauty business, like the world in general, is evolving at an alarming rate, and even some of the absolute "truths" that we preached a few years ago we now know are actually false! This unique book helps the potential patient stay abreast of the latest, safest, most effective practices and strategies by profiling the very experts who are developing them.

Some of the experts featured herein knew they were interested in the beauty business from the beginning, and some of us came to it by serendipity. After not being accepted to the Harvard Medical School, I whined to my mother about the injustice of the universe, only to be told that I should, to paraphrase, shut up and do something for someone else for a change. Two years in the Peace Corps in West Africa was fantastic but did nothing to dampen my interest in medicine, and even though my original acceptance letter from UCLA School of Medicine was eaten by Ghanaian goats, I managed to matriculate there anyway in 1976.

Convinced for several years that I was headed to family practice medicine, I noticed in my final year of medical school that surgeons tended to love their work, and I set out for five years of surgical training at the Massachusetts General Hospital. Surgery training only created more choices: cardiac surgery, vascular surgery, abdominal surgery, etc. In the end, I was utterly mesmerized by the freedom of plastic surgeons to operate anywhere in the body and to deal with impossible problems from the top of the head to the sole of the foot. I accepted a residency in plastic surgery at the Institute for Reconstructive Plastic Surgery at NYU in New York City and joined the faculty there in 1989. The early part of my career was focused on pediatric craniofacial surgery. The interest and expertise in cosmetic (also known as aesthetic) surgery developed because, as the years went by, that's what the patients who walked in my office wanted. So the beauty business found me, rather than the other way around.

When I was training I thought that I would learn to be good at all the procedures in plastic surgery. That was naïve. As the years go on, all successful plastic surgeons become more specialized. Modern-day patients demand subspecialty expertise, not a superficial knowledge of every topic. Beware the doctor who is an expert at everything!

The beauty industry has never been more complex and more dynamic. The search for new fillers, topical neurotoxins, and less invasive procedures to treat aging changes is proceeding at a staggering pace. Cosmetic surgery, once the domain of the rich and famous, is now accessible to all. Congratulations to Beth Buckley for tackling this fascinating field in such a unique and educational way; *Mastering Beauty* is a great contribution.

Dr. Charles Thorne

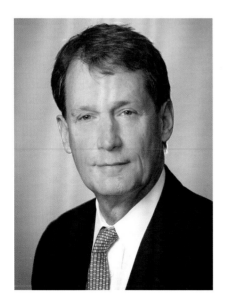

"Beauty is observing the graceful laughter of those you love."

Charles Thorne

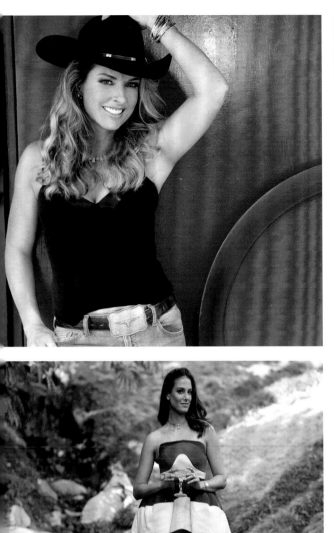
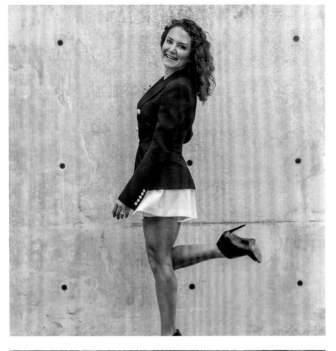
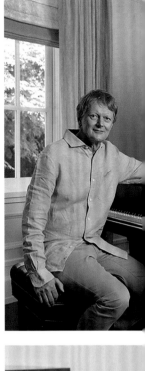
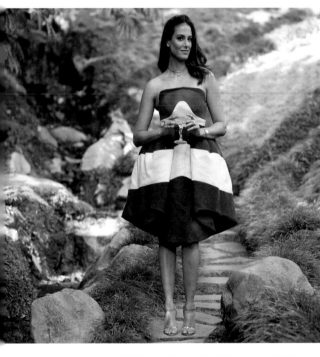
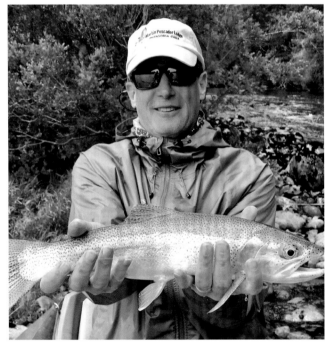
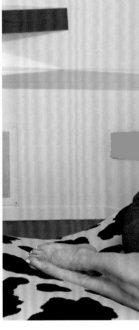
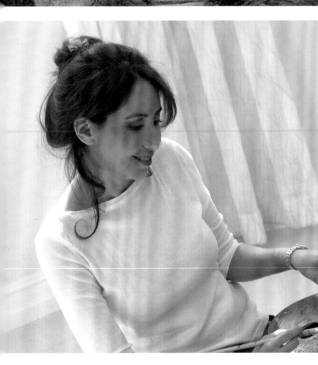
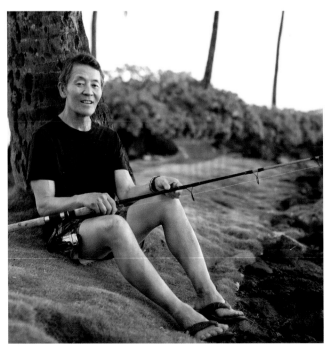
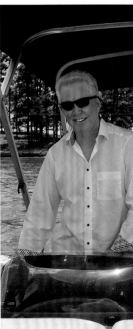

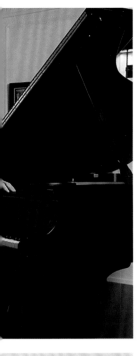
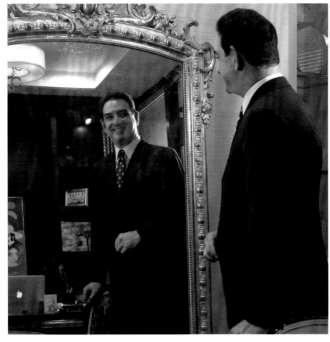
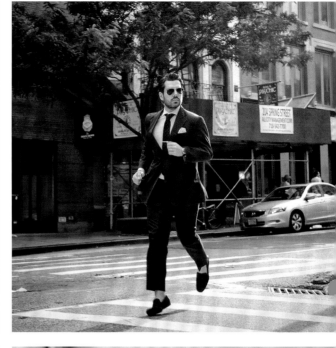
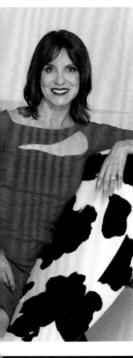
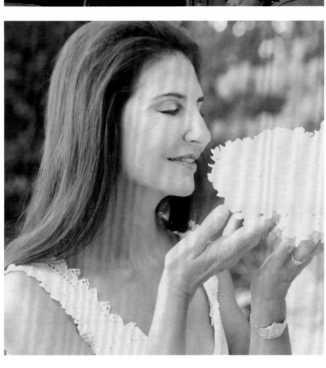
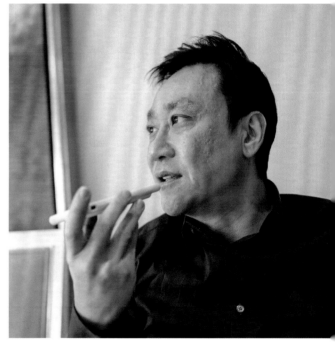
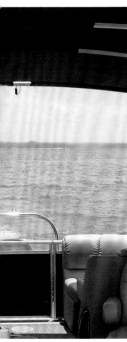
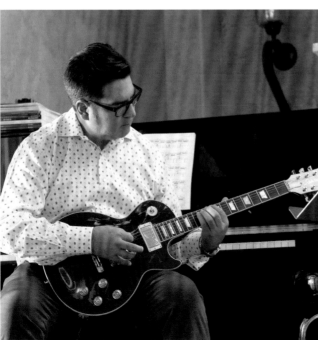
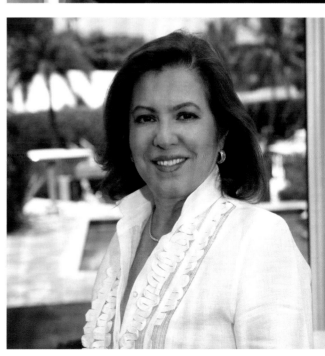

# INTRODUCTION

Beauty has been a fascination since the dawn of time. The human form was depicted on the walls of caves thousands of years ago, and it has been drawn, painted, and sculpted for centuries since. With modern advances in aesthetic procedures and treatments, maintaining a youthful, healthy appearance has become easier than ever before. Gone are the days when plastic surgery was only for the rich and famous, discussed exclusively among closest confidants. With the tremendous rise in the popularity of cosmetic surgery and aesthetic procedures, there has also been a significant increase in options when choosing the right treatment and the right provider. There is no shortage of information about aesthetics on the internet, though it's difficult to discern which source is best and most reliable. This landmark publication, *Mastering Beauty*, presents a fresh perspective on the latest and greatest products and procedures in the world of aesthetics, as seen through the eyes of some of the top aesthetic specialists in the United States and Canada.

If beauty is in the eye of the beholder, for anyone having cosmetic treatments and procedures, the most important beholding eye is that of the doctor performing those procedures. *Mastering Beauty* gives unique insight into a range of opinions from experts practicing a variety of specialties. This book provides a rare glimpse into the private lives, motivations, and influences shaping these masters' viewpoints. Every specialist contributing to *Mastering Beauty* has been vetted and meets the highest standard of expertise, skill, and ethical practices. All are board-certified doctors with many years of experience, each recognized and respected in their specialty. Despite sharing the highest qualifications in common, you will find that the opinions provided by these experts are often as unique as each of their backgrounds. What is consistent throughout *Mastering Beauty* is the doctors' dedication to providing honest, accurate information, and their commitment to patient safety.

Whether you're researching options for your own rejuvenation or simply curious about aesthetics, enjoy and trust the information shared by these doctors of cosmetic medicine as you embark on your own quest of *Mastering Beauty*.

Dr. Adam Rubinstein

"It is the transformation of the entire person on a very fundamental level, a renewing of their spirit and energy. This is the power of cosmetic surgery."

Tracy Pfeifer

"You want to find someone who's honest and also really good at what they do."
Charles Lee

# CHOOSING WISELY

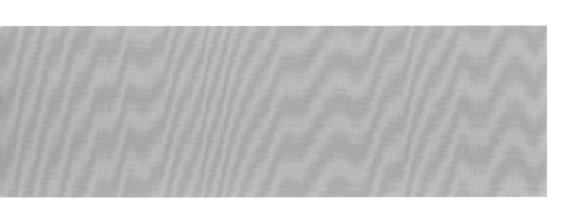

## WHEN SOMEONE'S LOOKING FOR A DOCTOR, HOW DO THEY KNOW WHEN THEY'VE FOUND ONE OF THE GREATS?

**Richard Warren:** There are great surgeons in all corners of the world, so it's not a question of geography. In any field of medicine, great doctors always have a passion for their work, which translates into constantly striving for perfection and continual improvement. Great doctors do their work with humility, and they usually have an obvious ability to connect with people. In the cosmetic field, that means a surgeon who has empathy for the patient's requests and who puts the patient's interests ahead of everything else. When it comes to the actual treatment, he will consider patient safety before anything else. He will explain things thoroughly, including the good and bad, and he will come up with a surgical solution that is customized. He may suggest several different approaches, because the knowledgeable surgeon will be familiar with a wide spectrum of possibilities. In the end, the great surgeon will want to do what is right for the patient, and that may involve recommending no surgery at all.

**Ashley Gordon:** When it's near impossible to get an appointment.

**Marta Rendon:** When they find a doctor who is a key opinion leader in their field and a caring physician. Doctors who publish, do research, and educate other doctors and patients are always on top of the latest trends and treatments. Of course the doctor should have great training and experience in their particular field.

**Adam Rubinstein:** Reputation carries a lot of weight. There will often be a few names you'll hear over and over again as you ask your friends for recommendations. But what's great for one person is not necessarily great for another. The main thing that makes a doctor "one of the greats" is that he or she is great when you have your visit in the office. The vibe you get can make all the difference in your confidence level and even in the end results.

**Tracy Pfeifer:** A "great" is someone who is experienced, consistently delivers beautiful results, cares about their patients as human beings, and is ethical. It is rare to find all these qualities in one person. I guess one could make the argument that caring about the patient does not matter as long as the doctor delivers good results and is ethical. But I include caring as part of being great because the patient's experience, which is better when they sense the doctor and staff care about them, is important. The positive benefits from experiencing "caring" should not be underestimated. How to know you've found a great? The doctor specializes in the procedure the patient is seeking. How to know a specialist? They did a fellowship in the area, and the majority of their practice is dedicated to the area. They have enough years of experience, 10 or more, to truly be experienced in a certain procedure. They are known for performing revisions of the procedure in question. Revision cases are often much harder than the primary procedure; many experienced doctors will not perform revisions of other doctors' surgeries because of how difficult they can be. They have published or presented on the topic. The staff and doctor project a warm and caring attitude. The before and after pictures have an aesthetic that matches that of the patient. The staff shows you average and good before and after photos—not every one is spectacular. This goes to honesty. Ethical practices will educate the patient and not pressure them to book at the initial visit. I am wary of doctors who are the first ones to engage in new marketing practices such as Snapchat from the operating room, as they may care more about their own publicity than the welfare of the patient.

**Clyde Ishii:** First of all, the patient needs to do some homework or research before just hoping he or she will find or stumble upon a great provider. The patient needs to find answers to the following questions: Is the doctor board certified, and if so, is the doctor's board recognized by the American Board of Medical Specialties? Is the procedure within the doctor's scope of training? Most states allow doctors to do any procedure in their office regardless of their training. In other words, as a plastic surgeon I can perform brain surgery in my office if the patient allows me to do so. However, I can't do brain surgery in a hospital because I'm not trained as a neurosurgeon. Hospital credentialing committees strictly limit practitioners to their scope of training. Therefore, the patient should ask the provider if he or she can perform the desired procedure in a hospital. This question will cut through the maze of confusion regarding board certification, proper training, etc. If the procedure will be done in the office setting, is that facility approved by one of the accepted credentialing organizations? If the procedure will be done under anesthesia other than pure local anesthesia or local anesthesia with light sedation, who will be doing the anesthesia? Is the anesthesiologist board certified?

The patient then needs to see the doctor in consultation and ask if he or she performs the procedure on a regular basis. What happens if there is a complication, and who will treat that complication? Ultimately, does the patient trust the doctor and feel comfortable moving forward?

**Sheila Nazarian:** I think knowing a loyal patient of the physician, who has gone to her for years and referred others with similar positive results, is the best way to know. But that is not possible for most people, so they search online and go to social media. Reviews are good but shouldn't be the only referral source. Before and after pictures and board certification in the actual field of practice should hold a lot of weight as well.

**Robyn Siperstein-Paul:** A great doctor makes the patient feel like they are the only patient of the day and they are receiving all the time and attention needed to achieve the desired outcome. My patients often ask, "How did you know what I wanted when I didn't even know until I saw what you did?" Great results will enable them to finally look like the more youthful person they feel like on the inside—not a different version of themselves, but the best version.

## HOW SHOULD A PATIENT GO ABOUT SELECTING A DOCTOR?

**Armando Soto:** I think of this as a multi-stage process:

*Step 1:* Assure yourself that the provider is board certified by one of the American Board of Medical Specialties' member boards.

*Step 2:* Ensure that any surgeon you are considering has privileges to perform the procedure in a good hospital. Having hospital privileges for the same procedure means that the provider has had to prove to a hospital's credentialing committee that they are well-trained and competent in its performance. Without this, you have no way of knowing whether their training in the procedure was real and comprehensive, as part of an accredited residency training program, rather than a weekend course taken in a hotel conference room.

*Step 3:* Read all of the provider's reviews and ask friends and other healthcare providers (your gynecologist, your dentist, etc.) about that provider. Weight should be given to providers with lots and lots of reviews, and I would always be a bit suspicious if the provider only has a few reviews, or if they are 100% positive. None of us can please everyone all of the time, and when you deal with the general public, there are going to be some crazies that cross your path from time to time. If a provider has many reviews, you will be able to get a good picture of the reality of their practice pattern and skills.

*Step 4:* Finally, and perhaps most importantly, you should focus carefully on their outcomes (before and after photos). This is, at the end of the day, "where the rubber meets the road." These photos represent our product, what—combined with the experience you are evaluating by reading reviews—you are actually paying for when you choose your surgeon. A provider should be able to show you multiple, not just a few, photos of excellent work.

If you've found a surgeon who is board certified by the appropriate specialty, who has hospital privileges in the procedure you are interested in, who has a long history of providing excellent experiences for patients (as evidenced by his or her reviews), and whose before and after gallery shows many examples of excellent, high-quality work, then you have truly found "one of the greats."

# CHOOSING WISELY

"On a daily basis, I have the privilege of helping people rejoice in looking fresher and healthier, reflecting the vibrancy and youth they feel on the inside."
Anna Petropoulos

## TELL-TALE SIGNS THAT A PATIENT HAS COME UPON A BAD DOCTOR AND SHOULD RUN?

**Robyn Siperstein-Paul:** The provider tells the patient what they should do instead of first listening to the patient's concerns and then pushes expensive products and procedures that the patient does not want or need.

**Tracy Pfeifer:** Before your first office visit, check for these red flags: 1. The doctor is not board certified in the area in which they are practicing. For example, a gynecologist performing liposuction. In order to be properly trained in liposuction, the doctor should be board certified by the American Board of Plastic Surgery. 2. The doctor does not have hospital privileges for the procedure they are performing. A hospital usually will not grant operating privileges for procedures for which the doctor is not properly trained. 3. The doctor operates from a facility that is not accredited. Such facilities may not meet basic safety standards. 4. The doctor performs operations without a board-certified anesthesiologist when almost everyone else uses an anesthesiologist. This is done to save money and does not put patient safety first.

5. A history of malpractice cases and/or settlements or sanctions by hospitals, medical boards, and medical societies. Red flags to look for during the in-office consultation: pressure to book the procedure the day of the consultation; reduced fees to book the day of the consultation; minimization of risks and complications or refusal to discuss them at all, or saying "don't worry, nothing ever happens"; failure to require medical clearance prior to a surgical procedure; dirty office environment; stressed or harried staff.

**Ashley Gordon:** The doctor's patients show obvious signs they've had work done: a face that doesn't move, over-processed skin, skin that's pulled too tight and/or over-filled. Unfortunately, more and more segments of society are embracing the "overdone" look, and those who seek it out almost see it as a status symbol of sorts. To make matters worse, there's no shortage of bad doctors who are willing to overtreat these patients.

**Armando Soto:** They are practicing outside of their training—for example, their residency was in ophthalmology but they are offering you liposuction, or they trained to become an ER doctor but they are offering you a breast augmentation.

They do not have hospital privileges to perform the procedure you want. They have few reviews. There are only a few photos available for review. Photos are blurry, out of focus, or poor quality. They spend a lot of energy telling you (on their website or in their ads) how great they are but provide little objective evidence of it.

**Richard Warren:** The vast majority of doctors are good people who really want to help. That's why they went into medicine in the first place. However, not all doctors are great, and there are some that a patient may wish to avoid. In cosmetic surgery, the outlying doctor may come across as being more interested in making himself happy than in making the patient happy. That might involve recommending only those procedures that the doctor knows how to do or wants to do, rather than what is best for the individual patient. The surgeon may seem inflexible, arrogant, and unwilling to answer certain questions. There may be a reluctance to discuss complications—for fear of discouraging the patient from proceeding. Patients should be wary of a surgeon who promises things that seem unrealistic.

**Sheila Nazarian:** People who try to oversell or say there is a special if you sign up that day would be red flags to me. Health-related procedures require time to decide what is best.

**Adam Rubinstein:** Great doctors don't need to extol their terrific qualifications to you during a consultation. Beware of the "hard sell" where you're reminded of how wonderful the doctor is and are pushed to commit immediately with a deposit. And from a safety perspective, if the doctor doesn't have hospital privileges to perform the procedure you're considering there's a good chance he or she is not a board-certified plastic surgeon. Always ask if you can have your procedure in a hospital, even if you're not really planning to do so.

**Marta Rendon:** Are they dismissive of your concerns? If so, it is best to steer clear. A good doctor will make sure you know they are interested and engaged. Are they consistently updating their own knowledge and pushing the boundaries to better serve the patient? Medicine is ever-evolving—if a doctor is stuck on outdated techniques and procedures, they are not putting in the effort to give the best possible service to their patients.

**Clyde Ishii:** The doctor is not properly trained to do the procedure. The doctor is evasive when answering questions. The doctor or staff is rude or pressures the patient to have the procedure.

"From anyone who claims to know everything, to have seen everything, and projects a "know-it-all" personality: run."
Charles Thorne

CHOOSING WISELY

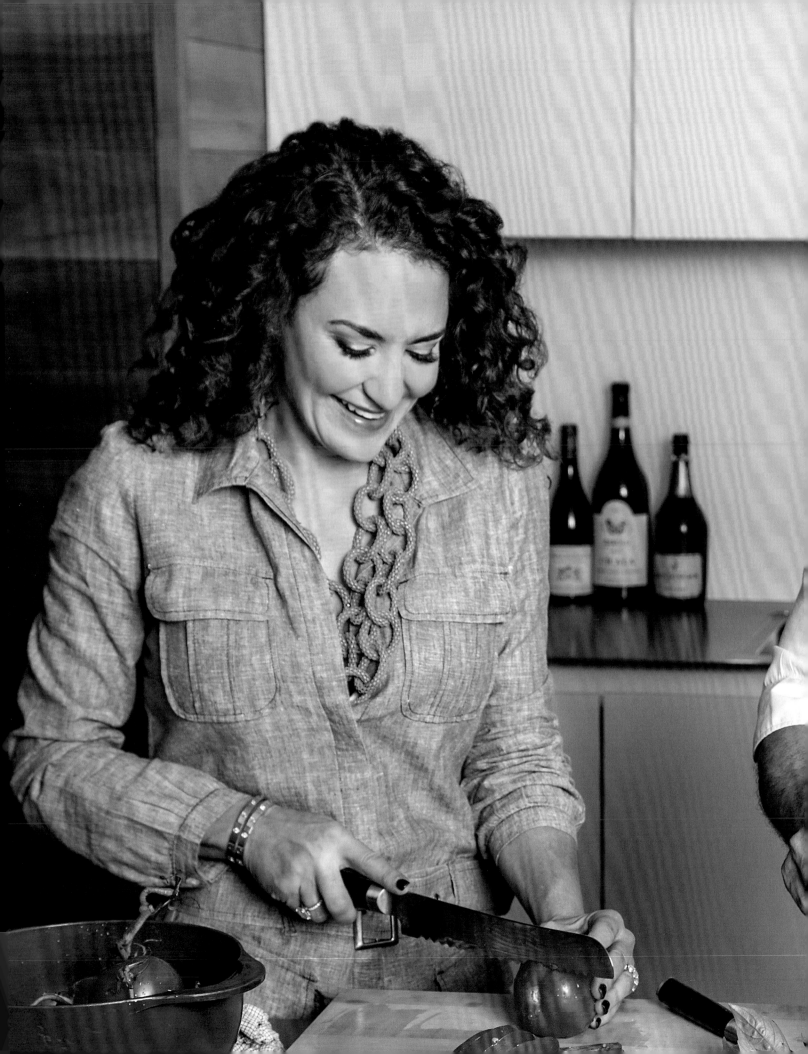

DR. ASHLEY GORDON

IN THE COURSE OF ASHLEY GORDON'S INTERNATIONAL food and wine experiences, she has realized that "great chefs and winemakers are cut from the same cloth as plastic surgeons. They're creative, technical, intense, meticulous, uncompromising, and relentless in their pursuit of delivering a great dish or vintage." Ashley aims to embody all of those characteristics through her pursuit of natural, beautiful results for her patients. "The best chefs and winemakers would never bastardize the ingredient or the grape by making it something that it's not; they elevate it and let it shine." So, too, does Ashley. She strives to enhance what's there without changing what makes it unique and special.

For Ashley, being able to carry out a variety of surgical procedures with exacting precision, fabulous results, and delighted patients isn't enough. As a perfectionist, she's always on the lookout for a better way—a more effective method to speed up the healing process, improve comfort before and after the procedure, minimize scar

## GREAT CHEFS AND WINEMAKERS ARE CUT FROM THE SAME CLOTH AS PLASTIC SURGEONS.

tissue, and maximize quality of care. She and her staff care about their patients' feelings as much as achieving the looks they desire. They ask questions and take the time to listen as patients share the depths of their experiences. When the team learned that most patients cite drains as the number one complaint in tummy tuck recovery, Ashley delved into the problem at hand—even though many in her industry didn't even acknowledge the problem, much less desire to change the long-held protocols—and discovered a way to avoid drains altogether in most cases. She turned an unthinkable idea into a best practice by listening and being emotionally invested enough to re-envision the possibilities.

Ashley cares deeply about how her patients feel throughout the process. She openly shares her experience of undergoing breast augmentation surgery many years ago. Her surgery did not go according to plan and the immediate results were not as she'd dreamed, so she was eager for a revision. Her healing process took longer than most, yet in the end she is very pleased. She is grateful for the uncomfortable experience and intense trust exercise that she had with her surgeon because it has made her a better doctor. Ashley knows what it's like to prepare for and recover from surgery, and she's all too familiar with the process of getting comfortable with the look and feel of larger breasts. She has empathy for what it's like to wonder, question, anticipate, heal, and keep wondering when the results will settle into their long-term look.

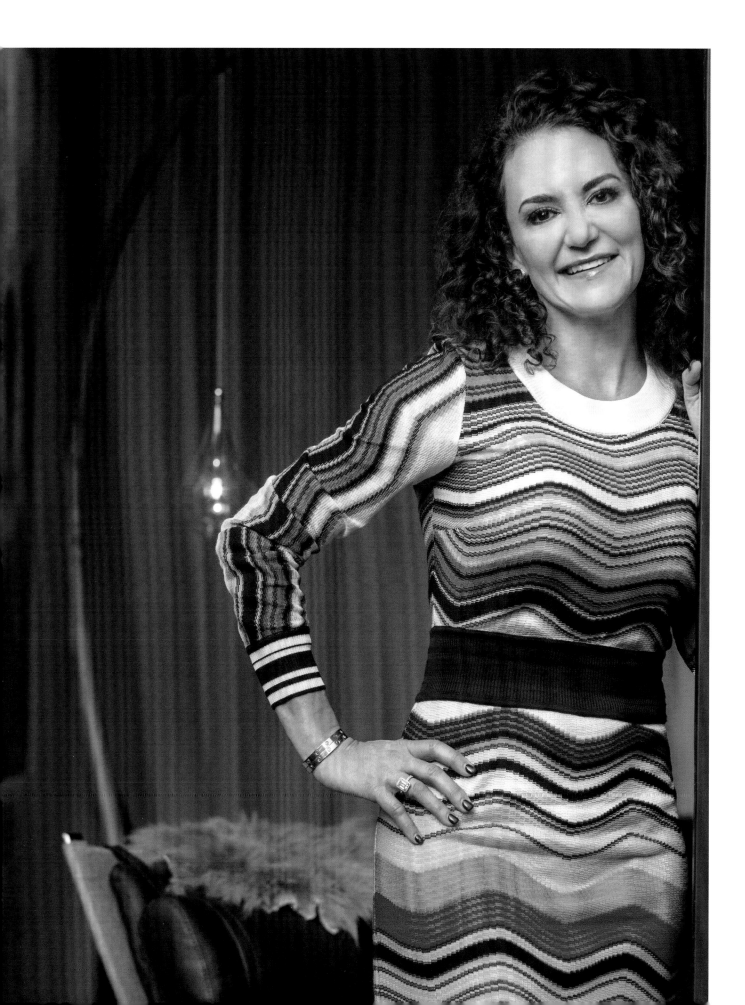

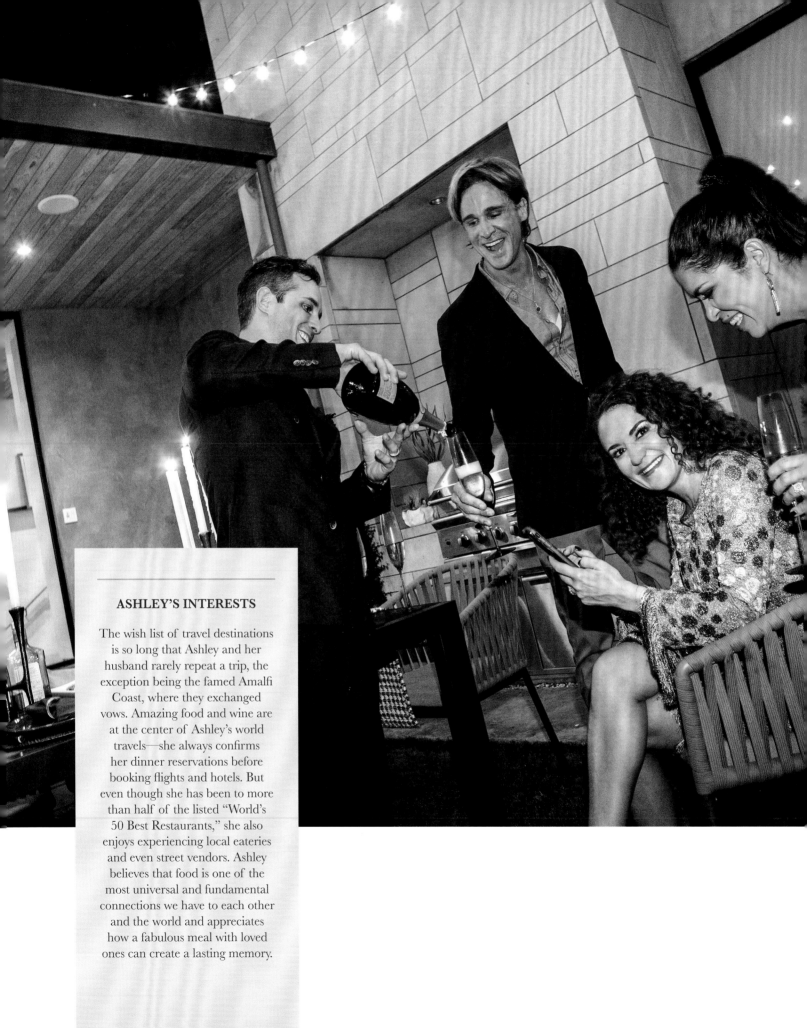

## ASHLEY'S INTERESTS

The wish list of travel destinations is so long that Ashley and her husband rarely repeat a trip, the exception being the famed Amalfi Coast, where they exchanged vows. Amazing food and wine are at the center of Ashley's world travels—she always confirms her dinner reservations before booking flights and hotels. But even though she has been to more than half of the listed "World's 50 Best Restaurants," she also enjoys experiencing local eateries and even street vendors. Ashley believes that food is one of the most universal and fundamental connections we have to each other and the world and appreciates how a fabulous meal with loved ones can create a lasting memory.

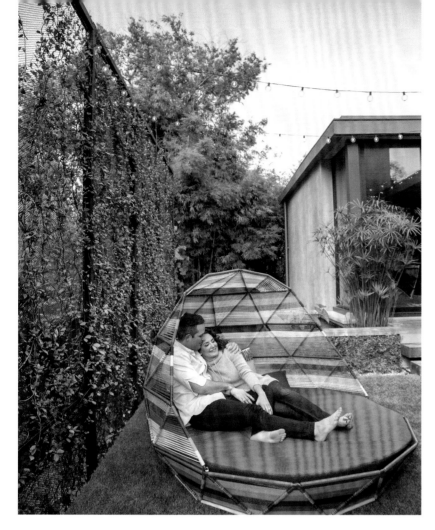

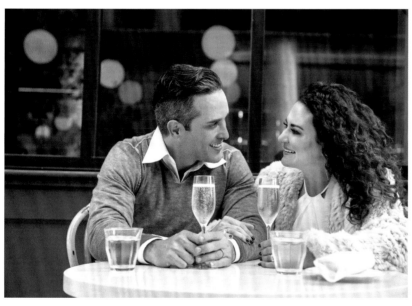

NOT SURPRISINGLY, ASHLEY IS extremely forthcoming with her patients about everything. In the case of breast augmentation, she and her patients work together to determine an ideal size and shape, yet everyone is aware that during surgery Ashley will do whatever she needs to do to achieve the best look possible. Figuring out the best placement and size, not to mention how the existing breast tissue will support the implants long term, can only be perfected once surgery is underway. A good portion of Ashley's patients come to her needing complex revisions after other doctors have performed breast augmentations, lifts, and reductions. These patients in particular appreciate the breadth of her experiences—personal and professional—and her thoughtful yet candid approach to medicine. Because of Ashley's policy of openness and honesty, she is uniquely able to take on the dual role of respected doctor and trusted girlfriend. Patients know that she'd never suggest something that she wouldn't choose for herself.

While breast enhancement procedures have undoubtedly become her specialty, Ashley is well-versed in a variety of procedures. Whether enhancing the face, the body, or something in between, she focuses on identifying the patient's best features and accentuating them. Certainly, she appreciates traditionally held philosophies on beauty, though she fully recognizes that perfect symmetry isn't for everyone. Sometimes slight asymmetry gives a patient's face interest, really great shadows, and the kind of depth that somehow conveys his or her personality; Ashley loves telling these lucky patients that they are beautiful just the way they are—and coming from a surgeon, it's high praise indeed. Many doctors take an additive approach—fillers, implants, makeup—yet Ashley likes to look at the full picture and employ a less-is-more philosophy. "When cosmetic surgery and even noninvasive procedures are done right," she says, "everyone will notice, yet no one will know."

"You've mastered beauty when you inspire others by unapologetically being yourself."
Ashley Gordon

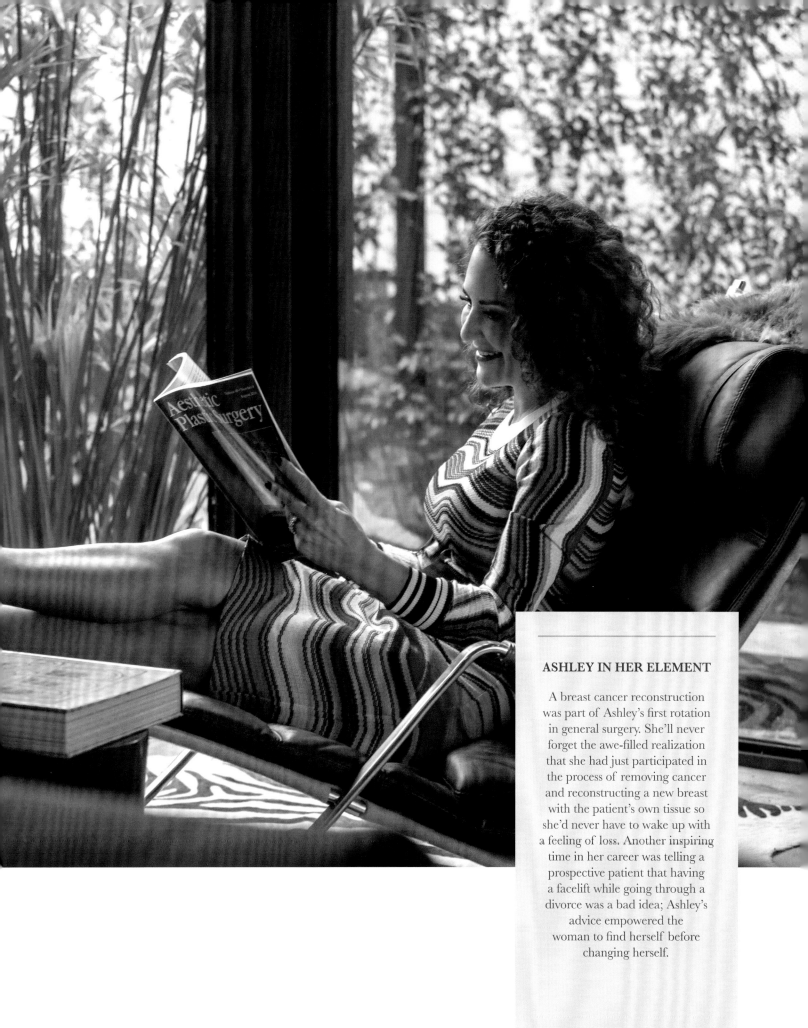

## ASHLEY IN HER ELEMENT

A breast cancer reconstruction was part of Ashley's first rotation in general surgery. She'll never forget the awe-filled realization that she had just participated in the process of removing cancer and reconstructing a new breast with the patient's own tissue so she'd never have to wake up with a feeling of loss. Another inspiring time in her career was telling a prospective patient that having a facelift while going through a divorce was a bad idea; Ashley's advice empowered the woman to find herself before changing herself.

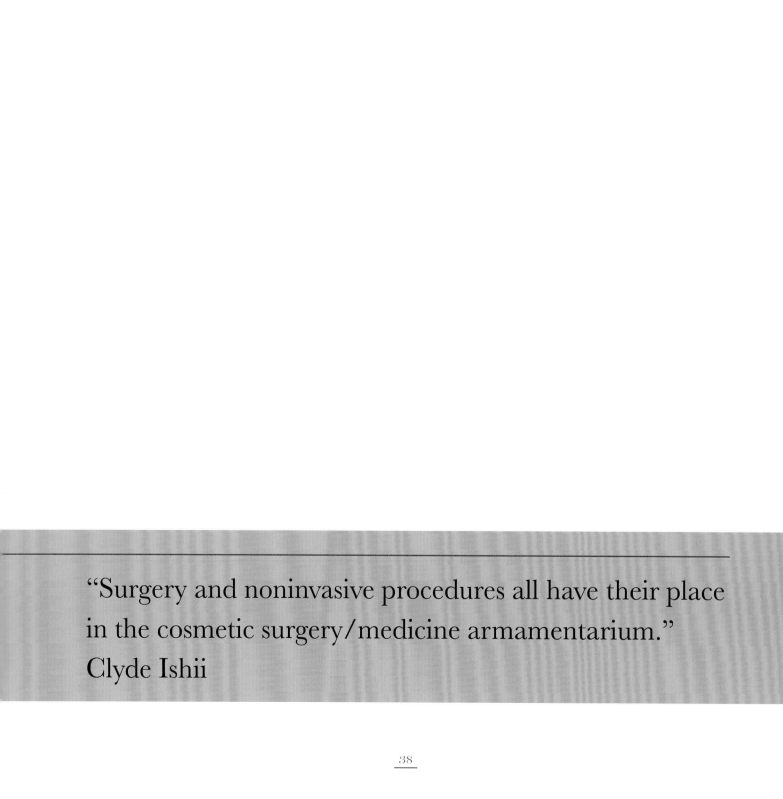

"Surgery and noninvasive procedures all have their place in the cosmetic surgery/medicine armamentarium."
Clyde Ishii

# SURGICAL OR NONINVASIVE

## HOW DO YOU KNOW WHEN A NONINVASIVE SOLUTION IS THE BEST CHOICE FOR YOUR PATIENT?

**Clyde Ishii:** Noninvasive treatments may be the best choice in the following situations: the patient has limited concerns and just wants a simple quick fix; the patient is on the younger side and is just starting to show the early signs of aging; the patient never wants to have cosmetic surgery but is open to noninvasive modalities; or the patient is a candidate for cosmetic surgery but is not ready to proceed from an emotional, financial, or scheduling standpoint.

**Ashley Gordon:** When the patient's tissues fit the criteria for a noninvasive treatment and the surgeon has the skill and technology to deliver a predictable, awesome result. Almost all patients would prefer a noninvasive option, but many are not great candidates. It's our responsibility to educate them on why they are or aren't and to be honest about how many noninvasive treatments they may need to even come close to a surgical result. For example, with some treatments, the cost and the downtime is actually less for a surgical procedure than it would be for five noninvasive treatments claiming only a few days of

downtime for each treatment. I've seen this time and time again with neck injections to dissolve fat versus submental liposuction, or fat freezing versus liposuction.

**Richard Warren:** Every surgical and nonsurgical intervention has its own specific indication. To give proper advice, plastic surgeons need a complete understanding about what the various surgical and nonsurgical interventions are and what they can do. In the end, it is really a matter of a surgeon taking the time to listen to a patient and formulate an appropriate treatment plan. If the best solution is nonsurgical, then that is what should be recommended.

**Charles Thorne:** Since surgeons do both invasive and noninvasive procedures, my bias is that surgeons are best equipped to make that judgment. If you only do noninvasive procedures then that's what you'll recommend. If you have a hammer, the whole world looks like a nail.

**Armando Soto:** This requires understanding both the anatomical changes that are causing the patient's concern and the desired outcome. Sometimes these decisions can be quite challenging, because patients will—at the time of their consultation—minimize their goals, hoping to undergo

a more minor procedure with reduced cost, recovery, and scarring. If I'm not careful to fully understand their dreams for their appearance, they may end up disappointed with their outcome. When there seems to be a good fit and harmony between the degree of improvement I know is possible through a noninvasive procedure and what the patient is hoping to achieve, I will discuss these options with them. I always emphasize that, even in 2018, the smaller the intervention, the more subtle the improvement will usually be.

## ETHICALLY, SHOULD ALL SURGEONS OFFER NONINVASIVE PROCEDURES?

**Armando Soto:** I think the important question is really a bit broader than this. I think that all ethical providers of aesthetic care should be able to offer a patient multiple options for the management of their problem, or have a referral relationship with someone who can.

**Ashley Gordon:** No. Surgeons should only offer services and procedures they truly believe in and are trained to perform. Many jump on the noninvasive bandwagon because patients are attracted to noninvasive options and because ancillary staff can perform many noninvasive procedures. Some unethical surgeons are drawn to these technologies because they are so-called moneymakers in the practice. If you are going to offer noninvasive procedures, you must have a passion for technology, be willing to spend a lot of time educating yourself on what devices actually work and why, and have a commitment to delivering predictable and great results.

**Richard Warren:** In the same way that most surgeons do not offer all the possible cosmetic operations, I don't think surgeons should necessarily offer all the noninvasive procedures. They may offer some of the noninvasive procedures, and they certainly need to understand what all these techniques can do so they can refer patients to the appropriate person who does them. In this era, very few doctors will have every laser, every skin-tightening machine, and every possible injectable, so interprofessional referral is common and expected.

**Clyde Ishii:** Surgeons should offer noninvasive treatments only if the patient is likely to have a satisfactory result. In patients with advanced facial aging, surgery is the better option because noninvasive procedures are not likely to make a significant difference. Patients must be counseled up front so they don't spend a lot of money on noninvasive procedures only to need cosmetic surgery when the noninvasive procedures fall short.

**Charles Thorne:** No. Of course not. But if they think a patient is best treated with a noninvasive procedure, they should recommend that the patient see someone who offers those treatments.

## HOW CAN PATIENTS CONSIDERING SURGERY PLAN FOR A POSITIVE EXPERIENCE?

**Armando Soto:** Often, patients are quite committed to a procedure that their extensive internet research has led them to believe is going to make them happy, even though (after an examination and consultation) I know the procedure they are asking me for is going to make them look funny or strange. They already know the operation they want—they just need to find someone to do it for them—and they have made this determination without an adequate understanding of how their starting anatomy and their desired appearance will affect the procedure chosen. This is a little like choosing a road out of town because you've read it's a smooth road with little traffic, but without consideration for whether or not it will take you where you want to go! The most important thing when planning your plastic surgery—other than choosing the best surgeon for you—is understanding that you should choose your experience and your outcome. I say it often: the most important three factors are not related to costs, scars, or recovery, although these are obviously very important. The most important three factors are:

who will be your surgeon; what experience you are likely to have in their practice; what is the outcome you are likely to achieve in their hands. If you choose the first properly, the other two will often follow; it is important to realize that having a good experience and the appearance you desired trump everything else.

**Jim Grotting:** Patients contemplating surgery should have a fully developed idea of what changes they think will make them happier with their appearance. Consultation with an expert will help guide them in their decision-making. Plastic surgeons should help educate and offer options. Not everyone wants to have all possible procedures to maximally move themselves in the direction of the ideal. Communication is the key to help patients feel fully informed and confident that they will have a positive experience.

## WHAT IMPORTANT QUESTIONS SHOULD PATIENTS ASK IN A CONSULTATION?

**Robyn Siperstein-Paul:** Ask if the doctor understands what your goals are and have him or her repeat these to you. To ensure your expectations will be met, it is also imperative that you ask if the

doctor believes the procedure will make you more attractive, more youthful, or both. I would also recommend asking if the doctor believes a particular procedure is the best course of action to achieve your desired results, or if there are other procedures the doctor recommends. Your expectations of the outcome and possible side effects as well as potential downtime that might be required post-procedure should be discussed candidly.

## HOW MANY PROCEDURES CAN BE PERFORMED SAFELY DURING ONE SESSION, AND WHICH ARE THE MOST COMPLEMENTARY?

**Charles Thorne:** Impossible to answer. There are some patients whose facelift takes 90 minutes and can be combined with several other procedures. There are other patients whose facelift will take four hours, which places a greater limitation on the concomitant procedures.

**Richard Warren:** The number of surgeries than can be done at once depends completely on the magnitude and nature of the procedures involved. Sometimes two operations cannot be done at the same time because one of them will interfere with the other. One example in my practice of noncomplementary procedures would be a rhinoplasty requiring nasal bone fracturing and lower eyelid surgery with orbital fat transposition. However, many operations are complementary, especially when they are done in the same anatomic zone. An example of a common complementary surgery is facial rejuvenation involving brow surgery, eyelid surgery, and a facelift. Other examples would be breast augmentation in conjunction with mastopexy. Perhaps the most common reason to avoid multiple surgeries in one session is the time involved. Excess surgical duration can be hard on a patient and may be associated with an increase in postoperative complications, such as infection and deep vein thrombosis.

**Clyde Ishii:** There is no specific limit on the number of procedures that can be performed safely in one sitting. Instead, the surgeon must think in terms of the physiologic burden or trauma from multiple procedures, and this must be balanced against the patient's preoperative health status. A patient with multiple significant medical problems is not a candidate for cosmetic surgery. On the other hand, a healthy younger patient has a deeper physiologic

reserve and can usually tolerate multiple procedures without difficulty if the surgeon takes into account operative time, blood loss, and other variables that affect recovery.

**Armando Soto:** This would really depend on the details of the patient's needs and the surgeon she chooses, in the sense that an operation that might take one surgeon three hours takes another four or five. The data shows that the risks of elective surgery really start to climb after about six hours, so the limit I hold myself to is procedures that I believe will take me about five hours, in order to have a bit of a safety cushion. If I know I can complete the combination of procedures in less than five hours—also taking into consideration the health of my patient—I'll say yes. If it's likely to take longer than five hours, I will explain that it is probably best to divide the procedures into two operations. As far as which are most complementary, this would depend highly on the details of my patient's anatomy and goals. Generally, "mommy makeover" procedures are amazingly positive transformations because the breast and tummy areas are the most affected by changes frequently experienced by women due to pregnancy and childbirth, and because they are on the same aspect of the body.

## HOW CAN PATIENTS AVOID GETTING ADDICTED TO COSMETIC TREATMENTS?

**Jim Grotting:** Addiction to cosmetic treatments is rare. Most patients who have realistic expectations will end up pleased with the choices they have made. However, the privilege of treating patients for aesthetic improvements also requires responsibility. It is essential that one evaluates and treats the whole patient and recognizes those individuals who may be expecting results that are life-changing or situation-changing. Those people often end up less satisfied. Of course, most plastic surgeons are very familiar with body dysmorphic disorder—those patients who focus on a particular body part and distort its imperfections only to transfer their concern to another body area once the original concern is addressed. These patients can never be satisfied and are made worse by repeated surgery. Treating patients with aesthetic concerns can be strong psychiatry with powerful outcomes, but conversely, treating the wrong patient can be destructive.

**Robyn Siperstein-Paul:** If you go to the right board-certified dermatologist, they should be able to create an annual treatment regimen for you that is realistic and includes a schedule for photofacials, fillers, neuromodulators, skincare, and other collagen stimulators to maintain your new look. This way you have a guide outlining the proper variety and cadence of treatments you should be getting to ensure you do not go overboard.

"Statistics show us that a minority of the population ever have cosmetic surgery. That means the ones who do are willing to undergo an elective operation with potential risks, side effects, and recovery time, in order to feel better about themselves. For the surgeon, it's an incredible privilege to be trusted that much, and it's a daunting responsibility we take very seriously."

Richard Warren

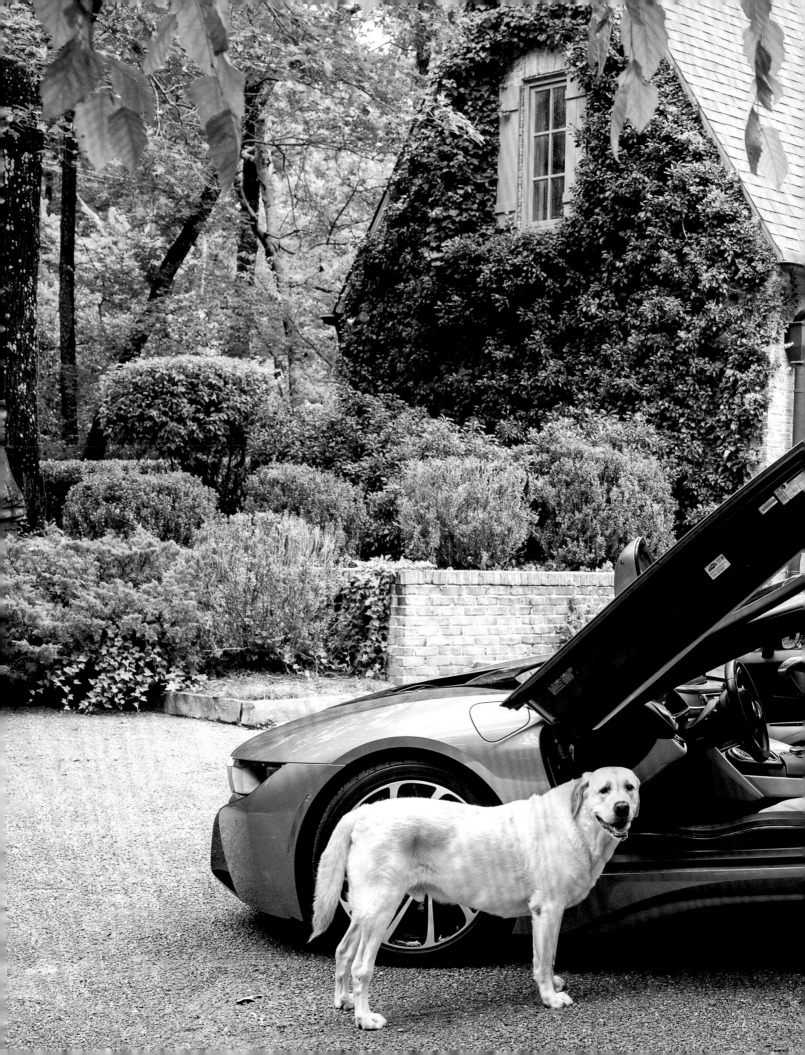

DR. JAMES GROTTING

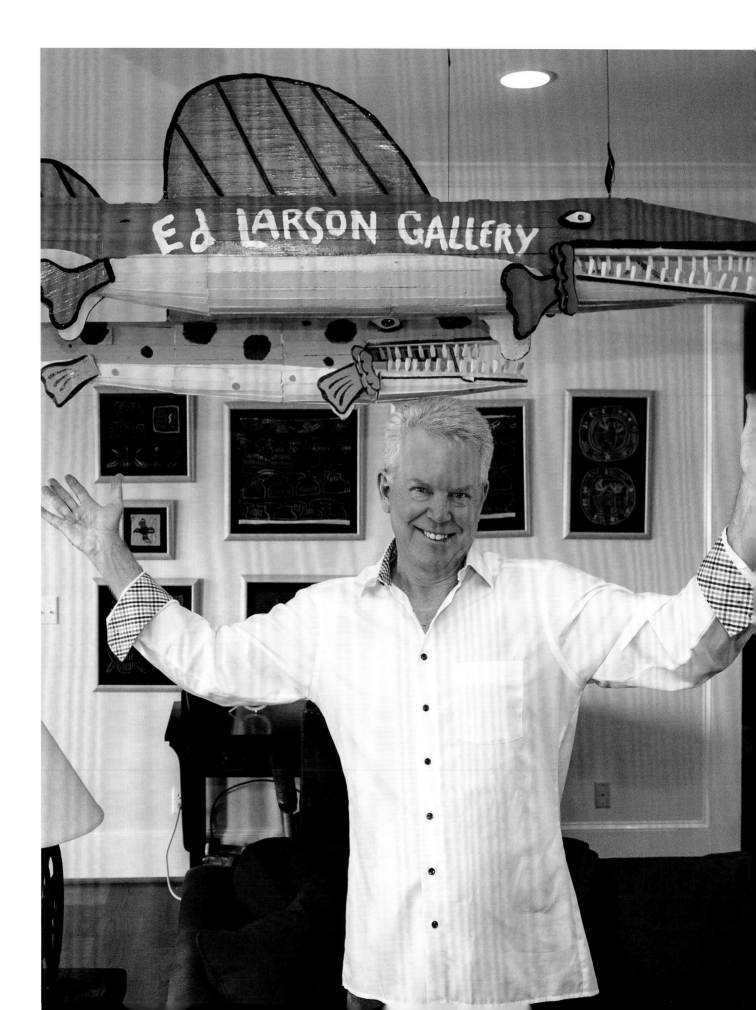

CINDERBLOCK HOSPITALS, OPEN WINDOWS, FLICKERING POWER—the adverse circumstances of performing philanthropic surgeries in third-world countries are memorable, to say the least. Yet it is within these incredibly humble settings that Jim Grotting has had some of the most profound moments of his life. And the rewards continue to trickle in decades later. One Filipino child who underwent a cleft palate repair to correct his speech grew up to receive a full scholarship for debate at a prominent Canadian university—and the young man sent a note of thanks to Jim, the doctor who changed the course of his life. Jim is inspired by how many times he has seen patients turn their toughest obstacles into their greatest successes.

Jim feels blessed to have become involved with charitable organizations like Operation Smile early in his career because they have given him such a healthy perspective. Along with helping underprivileged patients around the world, he has witnessed the power of professional collaboration

## PATIENTS CAN TURN THEIR TOUGHEST OBSTACLES INTO THEIR GREATEST SUCCESSES.

as doctors in sometimes-warring countries come together to effect positive change in their patients' lives and in the sociopolitical relationships of the entities they represent.

Jim has been careful to recreate the magic of his humanitarian service in his private practice by surrounding himself with a staff of professionals who put their heart and soul into their work. The people—his team and his patients— are what keep him coming into the office year after year.

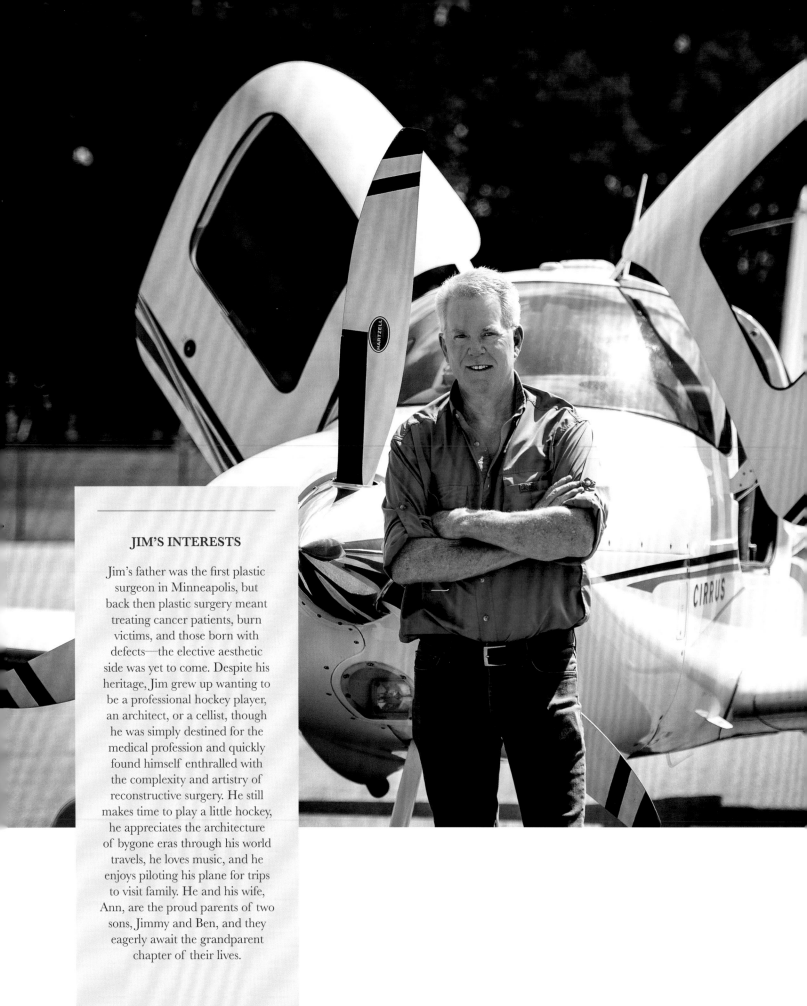

## JIM'S INTERESTS

Jim's father was the first plastic surgeon in Minneapolis, but back then plastic surgery meant treating cancer patients, burn victims, and those born with defects—the elective aesthetic side was yet to come. Despite his heritage, Jim grew up wanting to be a professional hockey player, an architect, or a cellist, though he was simply destined for the medical profession and quickly found himself enthralled with the complexity and artistry of reconstructive surgery. He still makes time to play a little hockey, he appreciates the architecture of bygone eras through his world travels, he loves music, and he enjoys piloting his plane for trips to visit family. He and his wife, Ann, are the proud parents of two sons, Jimmy and Ben, and they eagerly await the grandparent chapter of their lives.

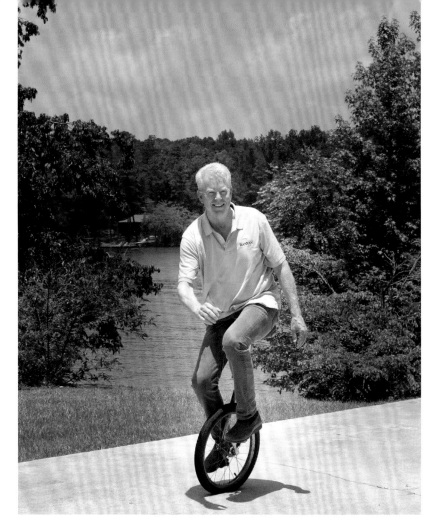

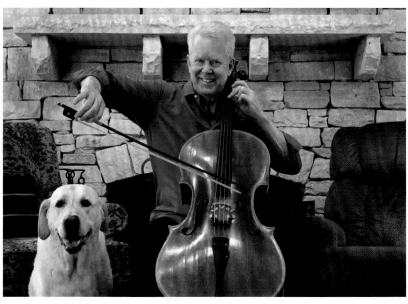

THE PATIENTS WITH WHOM Jim works are women, men, and children from all walks of life. Some seek his expertise for reconstructive or corrective surgeries, while others desire elective aesthetic procedures. Jim enjoys the consultation process more than most—he likes people and he appreciates the critical nature of this first interaction. In fact, he believes that the consultation is just as important as the actual treatment. During consultations, he respectfully yet candidly seeks to understand his patients' desires, why they want treatment, what they are willing to go through, and whether or not their mindset and self-perception will allow for happiness and a successful outcome. He is careful to accept only those patients who are motivated to live a healthy lifestyle—eating right, exercising, and caring for their skin—because they stand to benefit the most from his services.

Jim recognizes that the appreciation of beauty is hard-wired into us as human beings, and he feels privileged to possess the skill of restoring and delivering beauty. "Beauty is primal," he says. "It only takes a second to recognize what you find attractive, what you find truly beautiful, and the answer is different for everyone." Yet there are certain universals to beauty, and from the moment we are born, we subconsciously pick up on the cues—symmetry, proportion, skin texture. Even the most seasoned plastic surgeon may not be able to bestow the classic notions of beauty on every patient, but that isn't the goal. The goal is to enhance the existing look, make it more pleasing, more satisfying, more beautiful.

"It doesn't matter what the world thinks, plastic surgery is about changing how you see yourself."
Jim Grotting

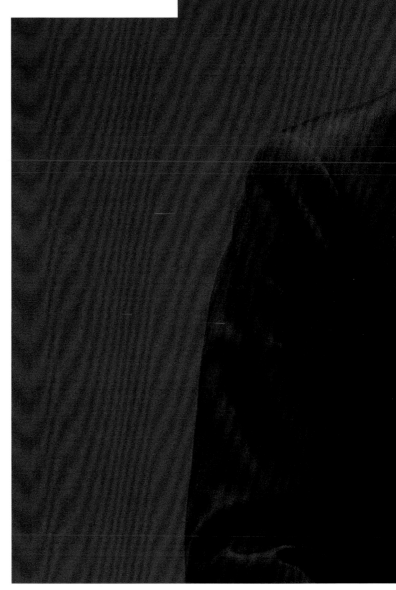

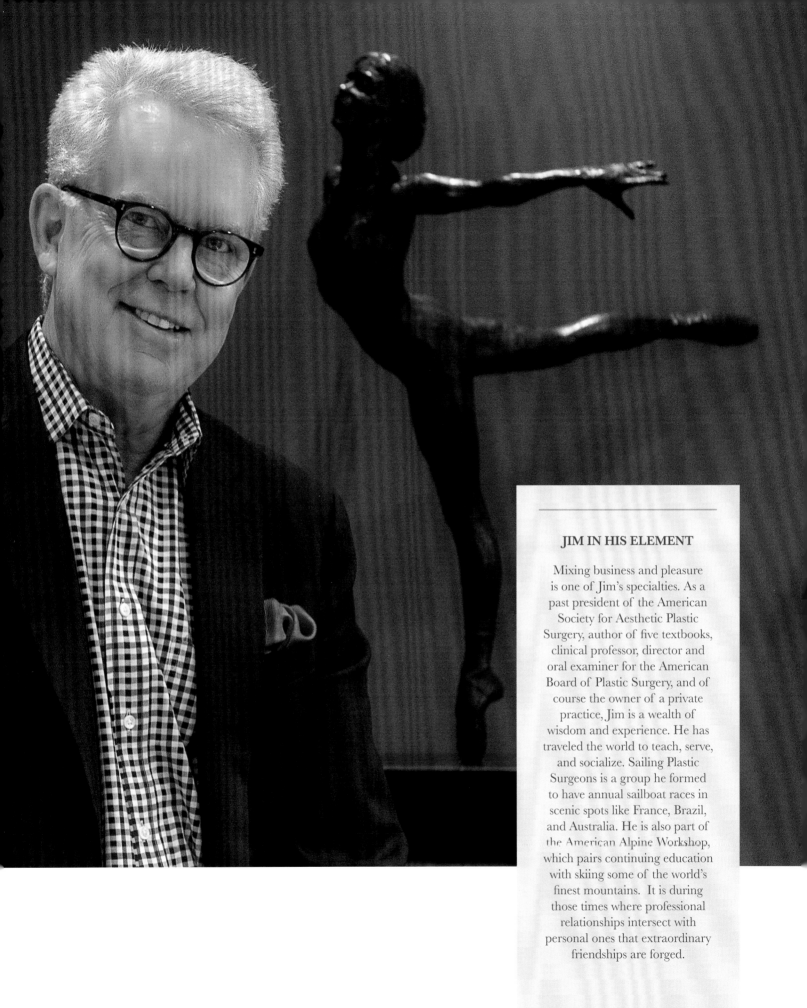

## JIM IN HIS ELEMENT

Mixing business and pleasure is one of Jim's specialties. As a past president of the American Society for Aesthetic Plastic Surgery, author of five textbooks, clinical professor, director and oral examiner for the American Board of Plastic Surgery, and of course the owner of a private practice, Jim is a wealth of wisdom and experience. He has traveled the world to teach, serve, and socialize. Sailing Plastic Surgeons is a group he formed to have annual sailboat races in scenic spots like France, Brazil, and Australia. He is also part of the American Alpine Workshop, which pairs continuing education with skiing some of the world's finest mountains. It is during those times where professional relationships intersect with personal ones that extraordinary friendships are forged.

"Those who are unqualified in this field are creating strange-looking people; they're distorting humanity and doing a disservice to mankind."
Anna Petropoulos

# INJECTABLES

## WHEN A PATIENT'S GYNECOLOGIST, DENTIST, AND DOCTOR ARE ALL ADMINISTERING INJECTABLES, HOW DOES THE PATIENT KNOW WHO TO TRUST?

**Adam Rubinstein:** You wouldn't go to an Italian restaurant and order egg foo yung, right? Why would you choose a gynecologist or dentist for cosmetic procedures? There is a reason certification in plastic surgery and dermatology exists. Doctors spend the better portion of their early life learning how to safely perform procedures and achieve good results. Research many options, confirm board certification, read reviews, and attend a few consultations. Not all doctors are the same.

**Armando Soto:** Yikes . . . I think that, whether you are talking about injectables or other "minor" procedures, it is important to see someone who can offer you many alternatives to that treatment. Otherwise you run the risk of choosing a treatment option simply because it is the only thing offered there. This is why I believe most patients will be best served by having aesthetic care performed only by board-certified plastic surgeons or dermatologists,

as ethical providers in these specialties would be best able to educate a patient about all options available.

**Sheila Nazarian:** Personally, I would want to be injected by someone who knows their anatomy and has trained in what they are performing. I would not trust someone working out of their scope of training.

**Richard Warren:** Practitioners in the "core" cosmetic specialties of plastic surgery, dermatology, and otolaryngology with facial plastics training will have had extensive residency and fellowship training over a period of five to seven years after medical school. This gives them a broader view of the cosmetic field and more scientific grounding than someone from another field who is self-taught or has learned to do injectables by taking a few courses. That's not to say that a doctor in another field can't learn to do injectables, but it is a case of "buyer beware." The odds of having a practitioner with a better background and, hopefully, better skills will be improved by going through one of the core cosmetic specialties.

**Tracy Pfeifer:** Well this is the big enchilada. Surgeons know anatomy inside and out, and because of this, some of us (plastics and facial plastics) are very good

injectors. We are not afraid to inject. On the other hand, some dermatologists are very good also. I would not recommend a dentist or gynecologist. The specialties that do the most research and training on injectables are plastic surgeons, dermatologists, and facial plastic surgeons. These are the three groups that I would trust. A consult with a surgeon who also does a lot of injectables never hurts. They know both the surgical and injectable options and will not hesitate to tell you which one or what combination is best.

**Charles Thorne:** The key is not just the credentials but how much experience the doctor has. Anyone can learn it. Most plastic surgeons have been doing injectables their whole careers while the others have just picked it up. In addition, injectables and all the associated anatomy and safety issues are a fundamental part of plastic surgery training.

**Marta Rendon:** It is about experience and results. More importantly, a doctor's background in education and training will provide the best benchmark for who to trust. In regards to injectables, a dermatologist has the upper hand in this matter, as training in this field enables the physician to determine if certain techniques fare better than others given the possibility of an underlying dermatological condition that a dentist or a gynecologist might not see or know of. Dermatologists and plastic surgeons are trained and have an in-depth knowledge of anatomy and facial aging, and their techniques and motor skills make them the most qualified to perform aesthetic procedures.

**Anna Petropoulos:** Take the example of building a house. There are different kinds of contractors. You would not choose a plumber to do your electrical work for obvious reasons; one cannot acquire the same amount of knowledge in a field without undergoing proper training. It's the same in medicine. After completion of medical school, it takes close to a decade of residency training and fellowships to gain the proper knowledge and experience to become a plastic surgeon. Why would you choose a doctor of a different specialty who learned a few details on a weekend course to do your aesthetic medical work? Patients should start with a board-certified specialist who has been properly trained not merely in the procedure but also in the art of aesthetics. And even that is not enough. One must also have a sense of harmony, natural proportions, and classic beauty. Those who have simply taken a

weekend injection course likely don't have training beyond the basic "how to," and there's no way to know about their aesthetic sense. Those who are unqualified in this field are creating strange-looking people; they're distorting humanity and doing a disservice to mankind.

**Ashley Gordon:** Patients need to do their homework and use common sense. If it seems weird to you—and it should—that your dentist and OB/GYN are now offering fillers, you should question what their motivations are and if they are even qualified to perform injections. I would hope my patients would question me if I decided to start offering pap smears or Invisalign®. These doctors' motivation is usually financial, and most haven't had any real training. The training is usually by the rep from the company. Also, those who provide these services will usually do so at a discounted rate, so buyer beware. You get what you pay for. I always explain to patients that they are not only paying for the product but also for my experience and skill in assessing what they need, choosing the correct product for them, and then injecting it in a safe, artistic, and skillful way. Also, if your injector looks overfilled, frozen, or "done," you will most likely leave the office looking that way too. Your face is your aesthetic.

INJECTABLES

## HOW DO YOU KNOW WHERE TO INJECT THE FILLERS?

**Ashley Gordon:** As plastic surgeons, we know the superficial and deep anatomy along with where the facial fat compartments are and which ones tend to age first. We operate in these layers and around these compartments all the time, so I think we have a distinct perspective when performing injections. We don't simply treat lines and wrinkles; we re-volumize to create more youthful contours and enhance features, rather than change them.

**Sheila Nazarian:** In residency training, we learn anatomy very well. We have also operated in these areas and seen them from the inside out. We know which muscles do what and what the consequence will be to paralyze one. We also know how the face ages with regard to skin, fat, and bone. That is how we know where to inject fillers.

**Clyde Ishii:** Fillers can be used to lift/add volume to tissues or directly fill wrinkles. A properly trained doctor will be knowledgeable in a variety of techniques. For instance, certain fillers can augment the cheekbone area and thereby also improve the adjacent nasolabial folds by the lift effect. On the other hand, the same filler in the cheekbone area can't lift tissues near the marionette lines, so these lines need direct injection with appropriate fillers.

## WHAT ARE THE LONG-TERM EFFECTS OF INJECTIONS?

**Sheila Nazarian:** Fillers can cause some collagen production, so over time it is possible that less filler will be needed if one starts in their 20s. There aren't really any downsides as long as you don't overdo it.

**Ashley Gordon:** We don't know all the long-term effects, and it depends on the filler; but when done judiciously and correctly, fillers can mitigate some of the gravitational descent of the face, and toxins certainly prevent deep wrinkles from forming.

**Clyde Ishii:** Most fillers today are made of hyaluronic acid and are temporary in nature. These fillers are metabolized by the body and have no long-term effects. Permanent fillers may have the following long-term effects: lumpiness, nodules, foreign body reaction, chronic infection, and cysts.

**Robyn Siperstein-Paul:** Anytime anything is injected into the skin, it stimulates the building of collagen and will have some positive, long-lasting effects.

"Do you want your injector to have taken a weekend course on fillers and injectable procedures, or would you rather they be an expert who attended medical school where they learned about your anatomy, completed a four-year residency where they learned how to properly inject and how to avoid complications, and then passed a national test to prove their knowledge?"
Robyn Siperstein-Paul

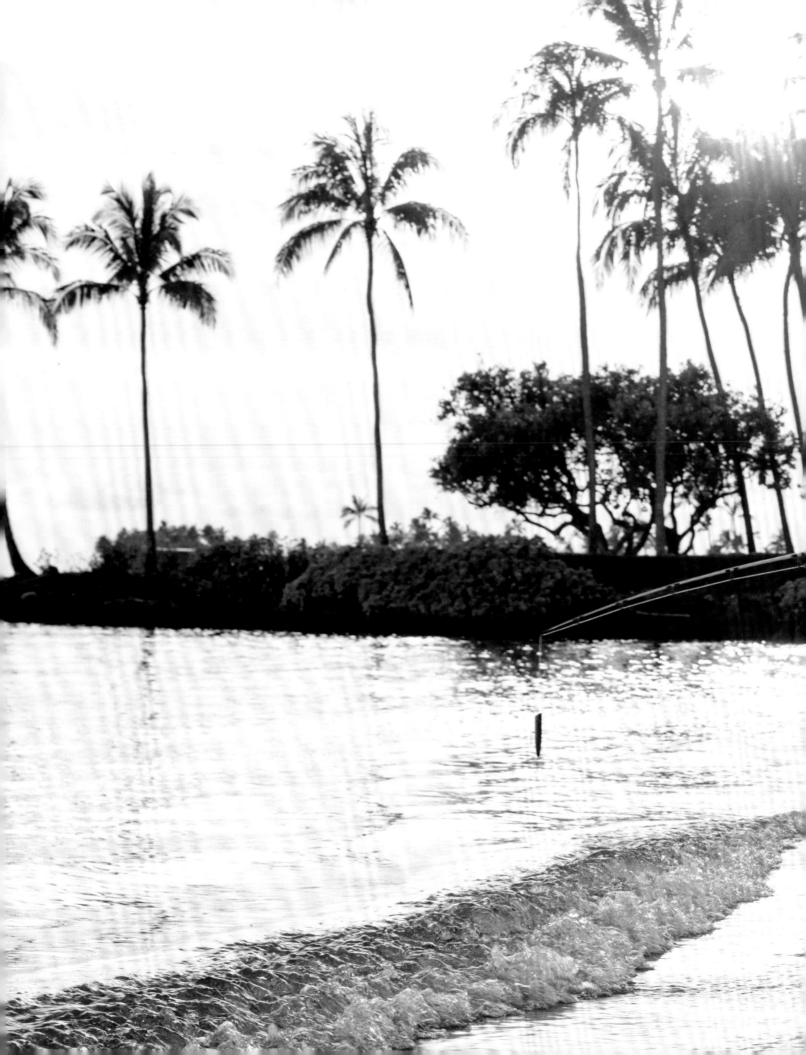

DR. CLYDE ISHII

B EFORE EACH PATIENT ENCOUNTER, CLYDE ISHII takes time to reflect on the significance of his role as a physician. He reminds himself, "This patient has entrusted me with his or her health and concerns. It is my honor to help in any way that I can." Each of his patients comes with a unique set of needs and wishes. Clyde feels privileged to have the skills to change the course of his patients' lives. He believes that we are all here on this earth to fulfill a unique purpose, and it is our responsibility to do our very best to take care of one another. With this overriding thought in mind, everything else falls into place.

## IT IS OUR RESPONSIBILITY TO DO OUR VERY BEST TO TAKE CARE OF ONE ANOTHER.

Clyde works hard to keep his life in balance, and this discipline makes him more effective with helping patients realize their vision of beauty. Perhaps his close proximity to the ocean and his intense love of nature provide the strength and inner peace to be present for his patients in such a meaningful way. The deep love that he has for his wife and children gives him the ability to treat everyone he meets like family.

Based in Hawaii, Clyde has a particularly diverse population of patients. Most of his aesthetic patients desire to improve their appearance while maintaining a natural look. He appreciates the profound cultural differences among his patients and is in tune with how to tailor his approach accordingly. This is especially true for his Asian patients who often desire more subtle enhancements. They seek an improved appearance that maintains their ethnicity. Some patients have an internal conflict of desiring change while still respecting their heritage.

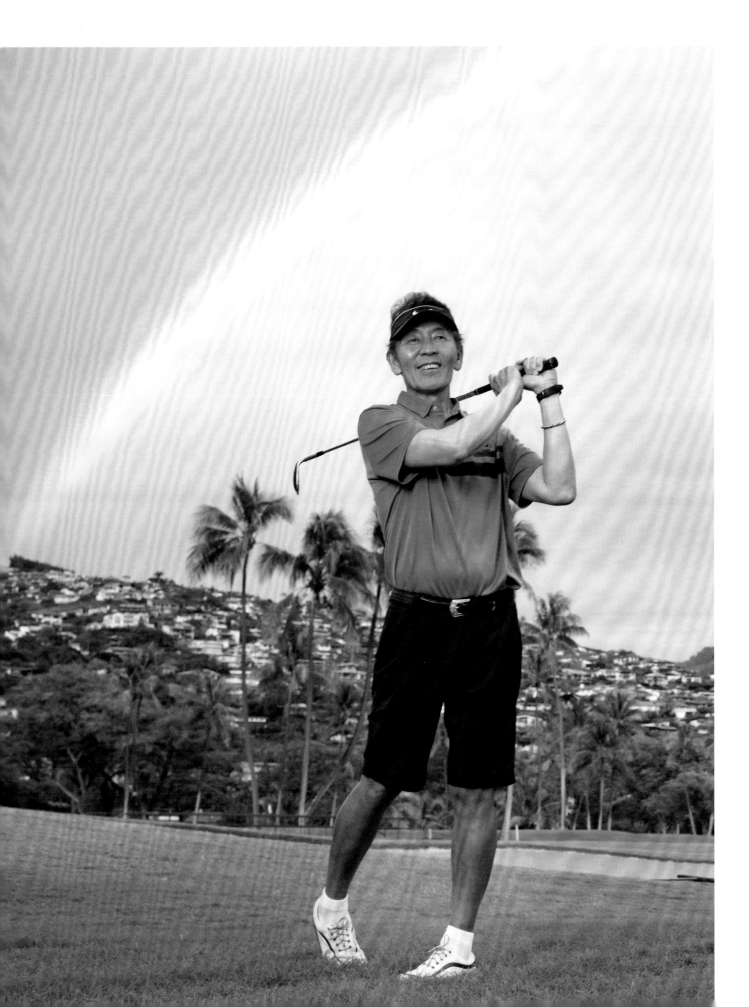

REGARDLESS OF CULTURAL ORIGIN, Clyde's patients share a commonality of desiring a look that is slightly more subdued and natural than those living in the continental United States. What might be popular in California and New York often makes its way to Hawaii several years later and is accepted in a toned-down version. Clyde likes his vantage point from the islands, seeing trends come and go, and then embracing only the most elegant and timeless enhancements for his patients.

Clyde spends the majority of his time performing elective cosmetic procedures; however, he still does a fair amount of breast reconstruction and hand surgery. He appreciates the diversity of the operations within his practice and the manner in which they complement one another. Knowledge acquired in reconstructive surgery is beneficial for cosmetic enhancement, and vice versa. "Starting out in practice, most plastic surgeons mainly do reconstructive surgery, treating patients with congenital anomalies, burns, traumatic defects, or the effects of cancer," he explains. "You build upon that foundation, and the knowledge gained is invaluable when working with people who appear perfectly normal yet desire enhancement of their appearance." Clyde acknowledges that cosmetic surgery can be extremely challenging, but the result is usually very gratifying for the patient and surgeon.

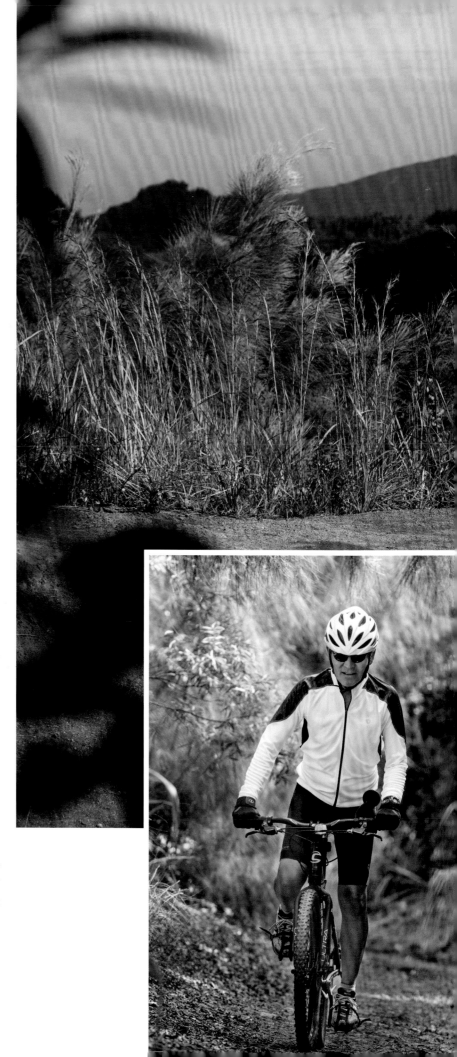

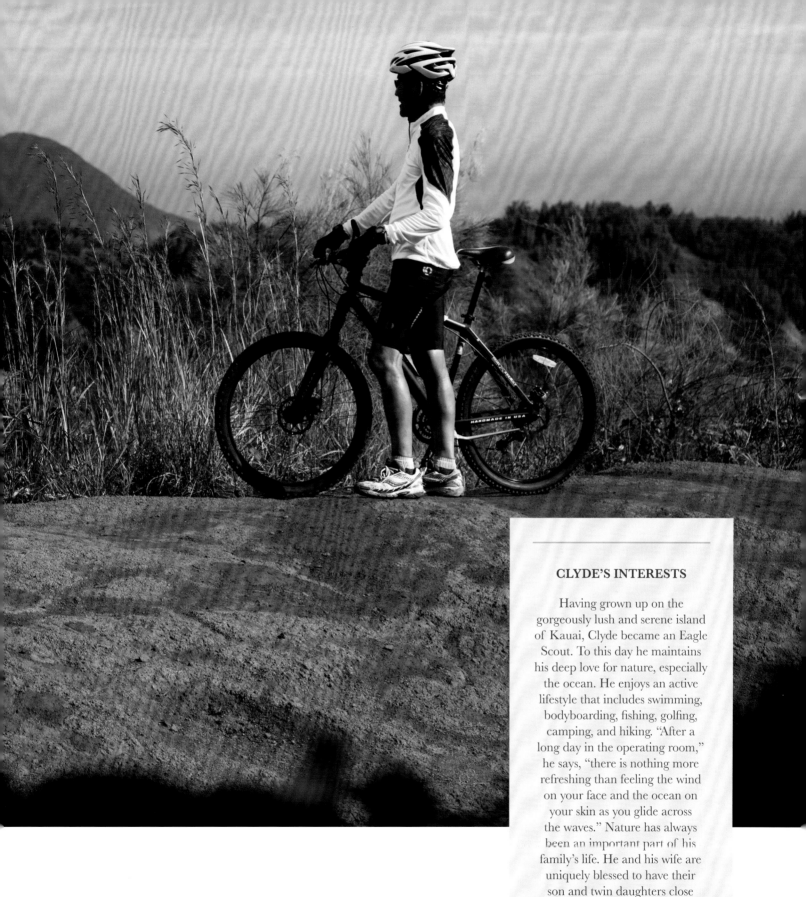

## CLYDE'S INTERESTS

Having grown up on the gorgeously lush and serene island of Kauai, Clyde became an Eagle Scout. To this day he maintains his deep love for nature, especially the ocean. He enjoys an active lifestyle that includes swimming, bodyboarding, fishing, golfing, camping, and hiking. "After a long day in the operating room," he says, "there is nothing more refreshing than feeling the wind on your face and the ocean on your skin as you glide across the waves." Nature has always been an important part of his family's life. He and his wife are uniquely blessed to have their son and twin daughters close by. Spending quality time with them and watching them flourish professionally and personally is their greatest joy.

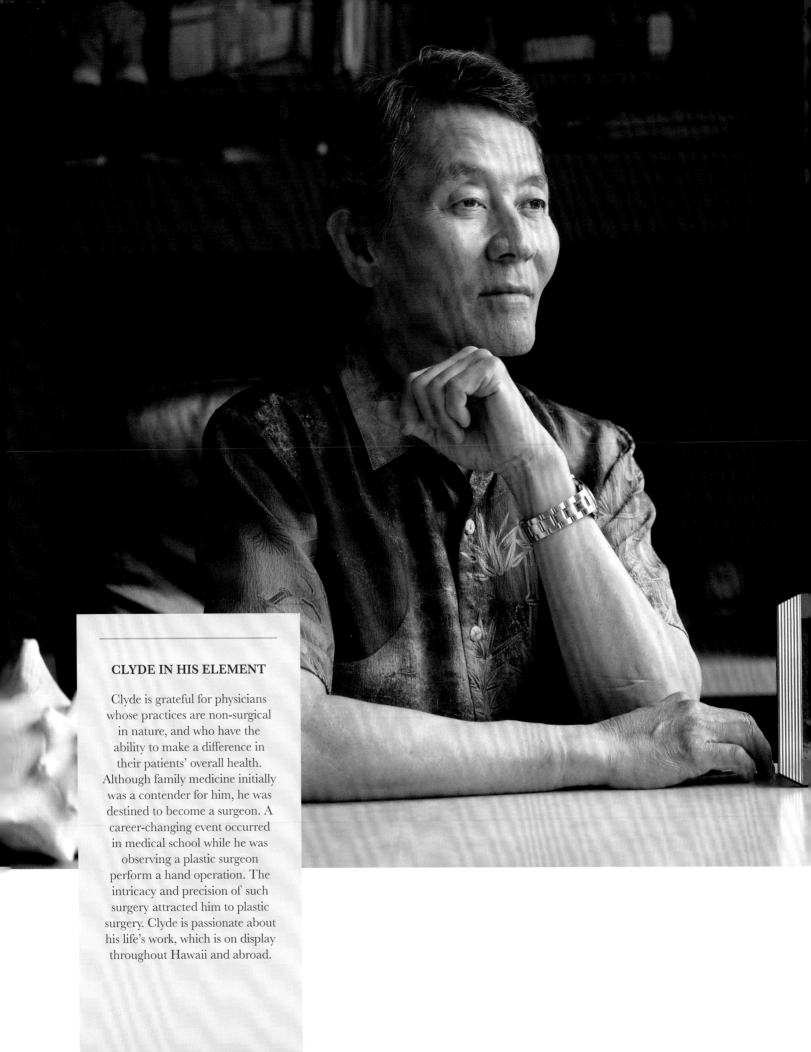

### CLYDE IN HIS ELEMENT

Clyde is grateful for physicians whose practices are non-surgical in nature, and who have the ability to make a difference in their patients' overall health. Although family medicine initially was a contender for him, he was destined to become a surgeon. A career-changing event occurred in medical school while he was observing a plastic surgeon perform a hand operation. The intricacy and precision of such surgery attracted him to plastic surgery. Clyde is passionate about his life's work, which is on display throughout Hawaii and abroad.

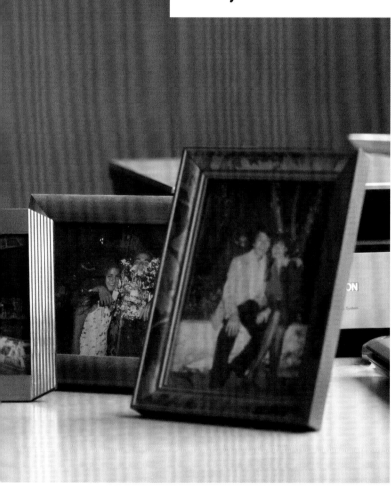

"Plastic surgery may sound very glamorous, but being a plastic surgeon is about helping people physically, emotionally, and psychologically."
Clyde Ishii

"I don't prefer the term anti-aging. It is inaccurate.
We all age; we can't be anti-aging.
But we need to age well."
Tracy Pfeifer

# STAYING YOUTHFUL

## HOW DOES THE COSMETIC INDUSTRY AND ITS ACCESSIBILITY AFFECT SOCIETAL VIEWS ON AGING?

**Ashley Gordon:** Our industries, along with Hollywood and celebrity culture, are the biggest influencers on how people view attractiveness. We know from various studies that attractive people earn more money, get hired sooner, get promotions more quickly, and are higher ranking in their companies compared to their less attractive counterparts. Attractive people also tend to be happier. It's great that our industry has so many options to help people look better, and therefore feel better about themselves. The confidence boost after surgery can be tremendous, and this permeates all areas of their lives. The downside is that more unrealistic expectations exist in society than ever before. People honestly think plastic surgeons have some sort of magic wand. Social media, various filter apps, and photo editing software contribute to a loss of distinction between reality and the idealized image that can be created.

**Sheila Nazarian:** Aesthetic procedures are becoming accessible to all, not just the rich and famous.

People want to feel good about themselves and see it as necessary to stay competitive with their younger peers. I think aging gracefully doesn't mean not doing anything. It means maintaining your skin, face, and body starting in your 20s.

**Marta Rendon:** Unfortunately a lot of the marketing is driven by the pharmaceutical companies that make these cosmetic products, and that in turn skews the perception of the consumer. Whichever company has the most attractive marketing campaigns tends to fare better. The results may not always be what the consumer envisioned.

**Robyn Siperstein-Paul:** Let's face it, we are so often judged on how we look, and now that we can do something about reversing the signs of aging, those who don't take action will be criticized. The upside is the advent of new innovations in anti-aging products and procedures that will ultimately lead to even better results with less pain and downtime.

**Tracy Pfeifer:** The cosmetic industry has opened people's eyes to the fact that as we age we do not need to inevitably totally deteriorate. This view is bolstered by a few very prominent celebrities who have aged very well, such as Christie Brinkley and Jane Fonda. Granted, they are beautiful to begin with, but seeing them look

terrific at an older age makes people think, well, maybe I can look and feel better as I get older. Both of them have had treatments, but they look natural. They look like the best version of themselves for their age, and that is the goal. Importantly, these two women have also exercised their entire lives and maintained their weight. Jane Fonda had an eating disorder, it's true. But neither had massive weight fluctuations, they avoided sugar (very destructive to our skin and internal organs), and I know Christie ate a lot of food rich in antioxidants.

**Clyde Ishii:** Direct-to-consumer marketing, media including reality TV, and social media all contribute to the public's appetite for cosmetic surgery. The result is that plastic surgery is much more mainstream than ever before, and there's no going back. The upside is that the public is much more aware of available treatments, and there is less social stigma for those undergoing cosmetic surgery. A prime example of this is gynecomastia, or male breast enlargement. It is estimated that one out of four men have some degree of breast enlargement. In the past, many men with this condition suffered emotional distress and lived with it. Today, many seek cosmetic surgery to correct this condition. Downside: Due to its popularity and portrayal in the media, cosmetic surgery is often considered frivolous and not real surgery. Patients need to understand that cosmetic surgery is real surgery and has real complications. Patients need to do their homework and seek treatment only from doctors with proper training. I ask my patients: "Would you fly in an airplane if you knew the pilot was not properly trained?"

**Anna Petropoulos:** This last generation is much more active, living longer. With 70 being the new 50, people want to look the way they feel and overcome the natural signs of aging. It is wonderful that cosmetic procedures are so accessible; however, patients must be aware of the dangers of going to the wrong place.

**Richard Warren:** Societal views on aging have shifted from an era when physical changes were considered inevitable and even celebrated to an era now where, for many people, aging is like an enemy to be defeated. This goes for health and fitness, as well as appearance. Many people do not want to grow old gracefully, and that has been driven by improved communication and wider exposure to all the procedures that are possible. For example, facelift surgery was once done virtually in secret, whereas now, anyone can watch it on a computer or on television, and most people know someone who has gone through it. People are aware of the procedures being done and they naturally wonder what these techniques will do for them. The downside is that aging is inevitable, and some people can become obsessed with the pursuit of interventions that ultimately are going to be defeated by Father Time. For some people, the more they see and learn about anti-aging procedures, the more they wish to pursue it. Inevitably, this can lead to unrealistic expectations and disappointment.

**Adam Rubinstein:** Certainly cosmetic surgery and aesthetic procedures have become more popular and more mainstream in the last decade or so. Surgery is not just for the rich and famous; it's more accessible than ever before. Consequently people have become more image conscious. Aging today is not what it was 20 years ago, and it will be different 20 years from now. Today, aging gracefully includes a little help looking fresh as time and gravity march on. There are lots of options when trying to look fresh, and age is not so important anymore when it comes to looking good. People are also more aware of the importance of taking care of yourself as you grow older. That combined with some maintenance and rejuvenating treatments can keep people looking great at any age.

## WHAT IS THE MODERN-DAY FOUNTAIN OF YOUTH, AND WHERE DO WE FIND IT?

**Charles Thorne:** Love. Let me know when you find something better.

**Ashley Gordon:** I know my answer is going to sound bizarre coming from a plastic surgeon, but despite all the great aesthetic treatment options we have, I firmly believe it starts on the inside with your attitude and with taking care of your body. Be nice, engage in regular exercise, choose a healthy diet, employ stress-reduction techniques, disconnect from your device, love deeply, and live your life with passion. These are the keys to maintaining youth, and of course, a little Botox when smile lines get too deep.

**Clyde Ishii:** There is no "fountain of youth," per se, but a healthy lifestyle is a great start. People who are interested in looking their best should start out with a healthy diet that is rich in antioxidants, maintain their ideal weight (avoid large fluctuations in weight), exercise regularly, adopt other measures to relieve stress, avoid cigarette smoke, drink alcohol in moderation, be sun smart (avoid repeated and prolonged exposure to the sun), stay well hydrated, and get at least 7–8 hours of sleep per night. Once a healthy lifestyle is achieved, the next step is good skin care. The skin care regimen should be tailored according to the patient's stage in life:
*Children:* Regular use of sunscreen and sunburn prevention
*Teens:* Appropriate acne care as needed and alpha hydroxy acids
*20s-30s:* Retinol or other Vitamin A product
*40s and older:* Antioxidants and retinoic acid

**Anna Petropoulos:** The fountain of youth is multifactorial. It starts with keeping our minds, bodies, and spirits healthy and being positive and joyous. Then we need to keep tabs on the five ways of aging: Botox® for our dynamic wrinkles, fillers for static wrinkles and volume restoration, radiofrequency to keep our skin tight, and fourth-generation stem cell cream to maintain our skin texture. The cream alone is the fountain of youth!

**Armando Soto:** The fountain of youth is the realization that life is short, and we should spend as much time as we can sharing experiences with those we love. It's found inside our own minds.

**Richard Warren:** Facial fat grafting comes close.

## WHAT DOES A MOMMY MAKEOVER ENTAIL, AND WHEN IS THE BEST TIME TO HAVE ONE?

**Clyde Ishii:** The mommy makeover usually entails cosmetic breast surgery (breast augmentation/lift) and an abdominoplasty (tummy tuck) but may also include liposuction in other areas. It can be done at any time after a woman has decided that she no longer desires to have future pregnancies.

**Armando Soto:** My definition of a mommy makeover is constantly expanding and becoming more fluid as we perfect more ways to restore a woman's body to its pre-pregnancy appearance and function. We used to think of a mommy makeover as consisting of breast augmentation with or without a lift (or vice versa) combined with a tummy tuck or liposuction. While these options are certainly still components often considered by women seeking mommy makeover procedures, they also usually include one or more of the following: vaginal rejuvenation; laser resurfacing of the face, neck, and décolletage; and tightening of skin in other areas.

**Ashley Gordon:** I prefer the term "pre-baby body." Women want to feel fit and sexy, and erase the damage that childbearing and breastfeeding did to their bodies. Traditional mommy makeovers just won't deliver the results most want. The most popular combo in my practice is a mastopexy/augmentation with an internal bra called GalaFORM® 3D, along with our signature Tummy Tuck 360™. The breasts are rejuvenated with a breast lift and a small to moderate augmentation, depending on how deflated the breasts are. The GalaFORM® 3D is a surgical mesh that is placed internally to support the soft tissues and maintain longer lasting results. This combined with our Tummy Tuck 360™, an abdominoplasty with circumferential trunk SAFELipo®, truly returns women to their pre-baby bodies. Many say that they look even better than they did before kids!

"I have great empathy for every mother who wants her tummy, nose, skin, and other uniquely affected areas to be as they once were. Through a combination of surgical and noninvasive procedures, we can restore our patients' bodies, confidence, and joy in life."
Jennifer Walden

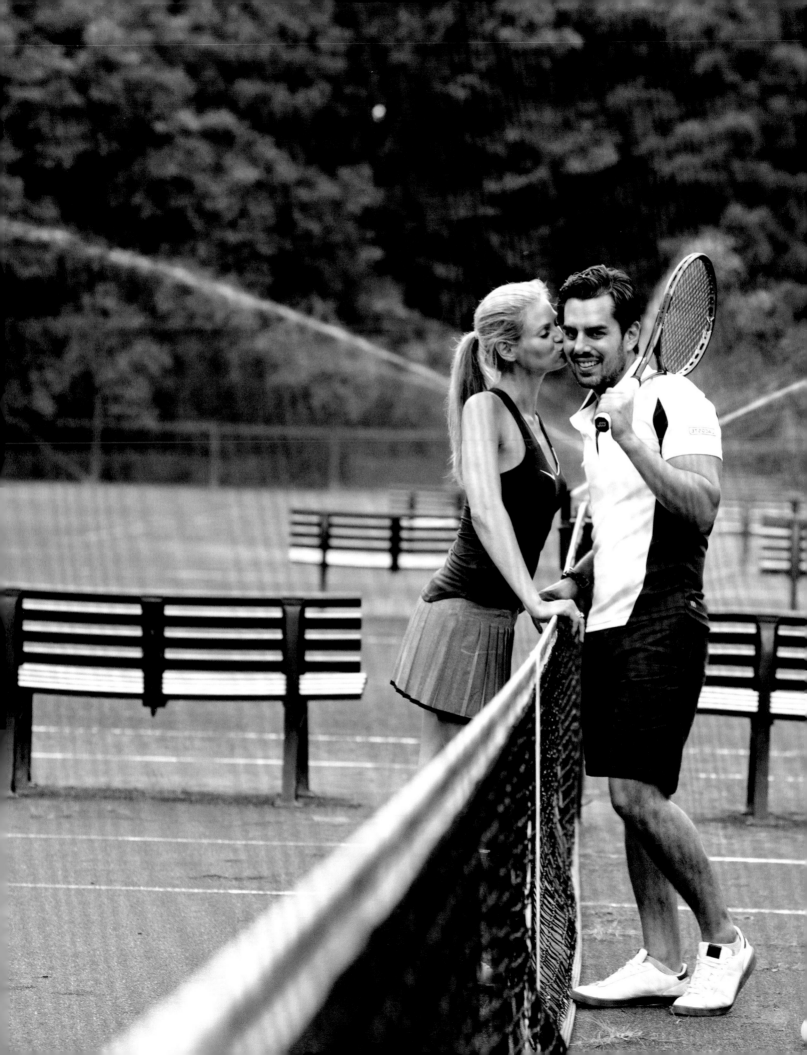

DR. JOHN KOUTSOYIANNIS

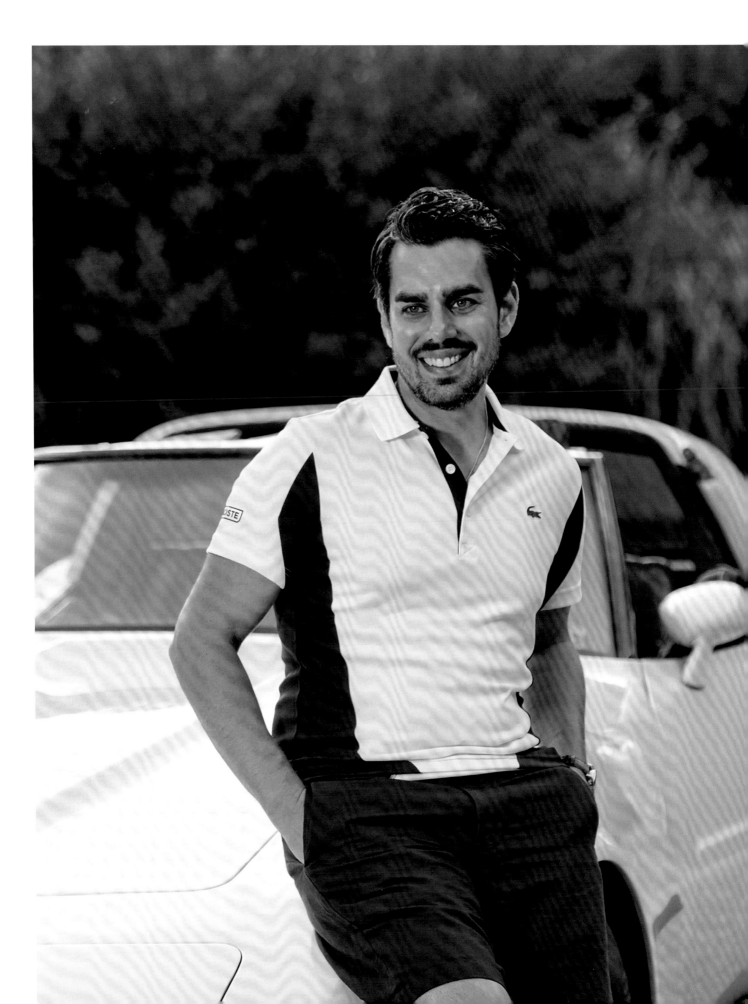

T HE FAINT TUNES OF THE ROLLING STONES drift through the corridors as John Koutsoyiannis designs people's smiles in his chic SoHo office. It's a creative process to be sure.

As a child, John enjoyed various forms of artistic expression. Painting wasn't necessarily his first choice, yet pottery always came naturally—he jokes that perhaps it's a deeply embedded characteristic of his Greek heritage. Today, he sculpts with porcelain to create smiles. John firmly believes that there's no such thing as a single ideal smile. Each smile should be as unique as the individual. "One person's perfect smile might look entirely wrong on someone else," he says. "It's about proportions and working with what's there to get the right look, a natural look."

It's certainly simpler to apply a cookie-cutter approach and give everyone the same full set of laminates that everyone else has—and goodness knows too many dentists do it—but John did not

## EACH SMILE SHOULD BE AS UNIQUE AS THE INDIVIDUAL.

become a dentist to do what's easy; he became a dentist to do what's right. "You don't always need a full set of laminates to change your smile. Sometimes it's two rather than 20. Sometimes the natural teeth simply need better positioning," he explains. His strong preference toward noninvasive solutions has created a loyal following and a clientele comprised entirely of referrals. And when laminates are the best route, he gives patients a full set of temporaries to try out for a while to make sure they look and feel just right, adjusts them as needed, and then uses them as blueprints for the artisan-crafted final product—everyone knows precisely what to expect.

JOHN ATTRACTS A FASCINATING mix of patients—from award-winning actors, world-famous designers, and models to diplomats, international CEOs, and local Manhattanites. Some patients only have to walk down the block to the office, while other patients travel many hours to see him. He enjoys treating so many different types of people, and he especially loves when they get involved in the design of their smile. Perhaps the best part of working with such patients is that they know his work and they completely trust his technical abilities and his creative sensibilities. They know he will make them more beautiful.

John has a thorough analytical process for analyzing the nuances of achieving someone's ideal smile—and he always goes through the steps—but truth be told, his sense of what's beautiful is so much a part of him at this point that the magic just sort of happens.

One of his most memorable patients, a diplomat, broke a tooth between his flight from Berlin to Moscow. Instead of embarking on his meetings, the man decided to fly all the way to New York to see John, who made a permanent tooth—an exact replica of what was there—in about an hour, and then the man jetted back across the pond. Needless to say, John's office is decked out with the best technology available. He loves the creative freedom this affords.

Changing people's smiles can change their lives. John had one patient whose teeth were

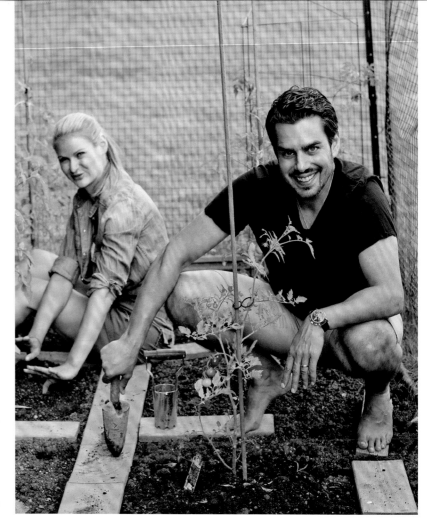

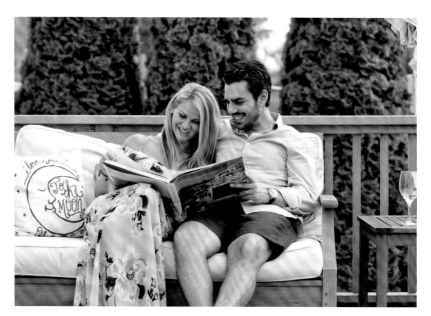

stained beyond belief from poor dentistry overseas. He reconstructed her smile and gave her more confidence than she'd ever known. It changed the way she carried herself—she was asked out by more men than ever before, and within a year, she met the love of her life and started a family. Being the catalyst for improving people's looks and lives is the noble quest that keeps John excited and engaged each day.

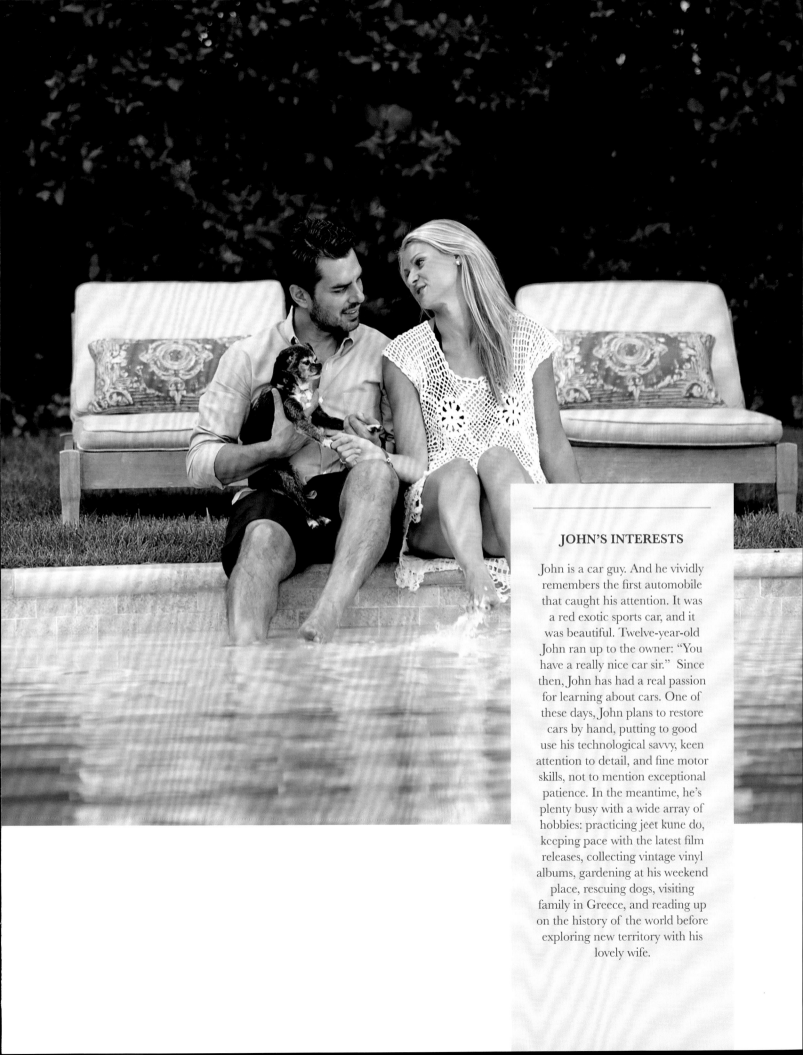

## JOHN'S INTERESTS

John is a car guy. And he vividly remembers the first automobile that caught his attention. It was a red exotic sports car, and it was beautiful. Twelve-year-old John ran up to the owner: "You have a really nice car sir." Since then, John has had a real passion for learning about cars. One of these days, John plans to restore cars by hand, putting to good use his technological savvy, keen attention to detail, and fine motor skills, not to mention exceptional patience. In the meantime, he's plenty busy with a wide array of hobbies: practicing jeet kune do, keeping pace with the latest film releases, collecting vintage vinyl albums, gardening at his weekend place, rescuing dogs, visiting family in Greece, and reading up on the history of the world before exploring new territory with his lovely wife.

"Going with your creative intuition always yields better results than following the textbook formula, because the most beautiful smiles are unique to the individual; they're human; they're perfect in their slight imperfection."
John Koutsoyiannis

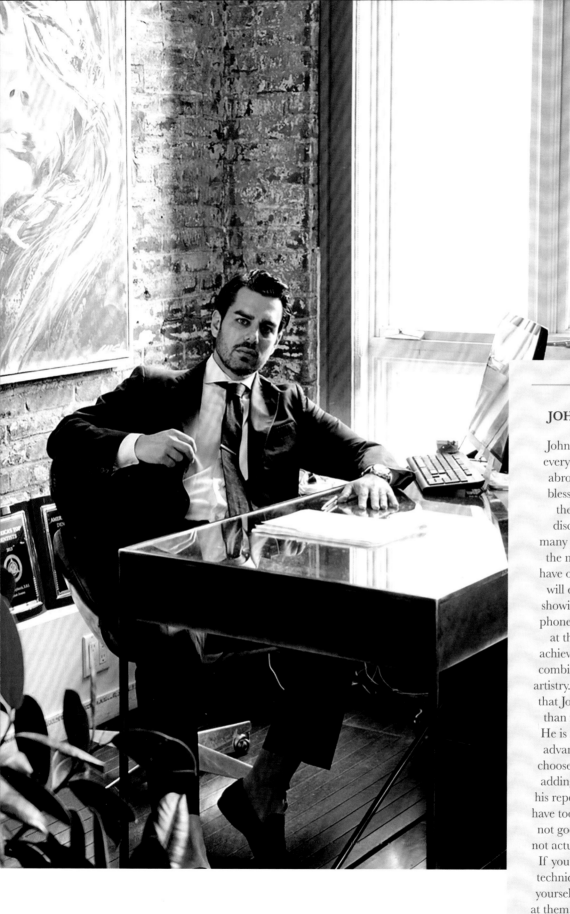

## JOHN IN HIS ELEMENT

John takes his work with him everywhere he goes. Traveling abroad reminds him of how blessed he is to practice with the latest technology and discriminating patients. In many parts of the world, where the norm is having teeth that have obviously been fixed, John will explain his profession by showing people pictures on his phone—they're always amazed at the natural aesthetic. He achieves these results through a combination of technology and artistry. Virtually every procedure that John does today is different than it was only 10 years ago. He is inspired by the continual advancements in his field and chooses wisely when it comes to adding tools and techniques to his repertoire. He shares, "If you have too many gadgets and you're not good at any of them, you're not actually helping your patients If you have your core tools and techniques and you really throw yourself into becoming a master at them, you can do anything, and you can do it at the highest level. You build on that knowledge, and that's how you grow."

"Some of what you'll find is truthful and very helpful, while other things might be bald-faced lies and deceptions."
Adam Rubinstein

# SOCIAL MEDIA

## WHAT SHOULD PROSPECTIVE PATIENTS LOOK FOR IN A DOCTOR'S SOCIAL MEDIA PRESENCE?

**Ashley Gordon:** Content that's educational, ethical, and fun! I think social media can be a great place to learn about the personality of the doctor and the practice, but the content should be informative and always presented in a professional manner. I've seen too many Snapchat videos where the surgeon seems more concerned with how he looks in the video than with his patient on the operating room table. The potential distraction of filming and posting in the operating room are of particular concern to me, along with concerns for patient privacy. Once it's posted, it's out there forever!

**Marta Rendon:** Social media allows a doctor to engage with patients on an ongoing basis days to months after the visit. This is also an incredible opportunity to remain directly connected with the consumers and give them an idea of what they can expect if they have not visited the office. Are they focused on academics or cosmetics? Do they provide information about what is going on with their staff? Are they constantly improving their environment?

**Charles Thorne:** If he or she has a lot of time for social media, he or she may not be the expert portrayed.

**Tracy Pfeifer:** If someone does not have a social media presence, don't count them out. Some of the best surgeons I know with great results and years of experience have no social media presence. A lot of people with a large social media presence have poor results and/or low ethical standards. On the other hand, social media can be a great way to further educate the public and let prospective patients know that the doctor exists. Look for people who are commenting on current topics in plastic surgery. Look for someone with an up-to-date blog that the doctor writes or approves—this shows an intent to educate and inform, as opposed to self-promotion. I think participating on Instagram shows the doctor is up-to-date, but the posts do not need to be graphic. Similarly, a business Facebook page shows the practice is modern, and it is a good vehicle for patients to stay current on what the practice and doctor are doing. I am not a big fan of Snapchat as, at the moment, the people who are very active on it are more self-promoters than educators.

**Sheila Nazarian:** Social media is fun, but before going to any doctor, call that doctor's particular medical field's society and make sure that doctor is actually trained in the procedures they are offering! So important.

**Armando Soto:** I think the most important question you should ask yourself as you review social media is, "Would I want that person doing surgery on me?" Understanding that surgery is a long series of small decisions, you want to be sure that the person you choose is someone who will make those decisions in a way that is in your best interests—and not because they might provide the most drama or entertainment value, or because they will look good in a video. I personally am very concerned about all of the video being shot in operating rooms—not because it isn't educational, or entertaining, and I do think that this medium has a role—but because of the distraction it creates. I want to always give my patient my very best, and I don't want to have the distraction of thinking about how we look on the video or what I'm saying to the camera.

**Clyde Ishii:** Try to determine if the doctor on social media is properly trained to do the procedure. Remember, social media is unregulated, so anyone can make a post and claim to be an expert in plastic surgery. The doctor's credentials can be cross checked against regulatory agencies.

**Adam Rubinstein:** Social media is one of many resources patients should use to research a doctor. Typically their style, knowledge, and communication skills will come through in social media, though things can be deceiving. Be careful about before and after results. A lot of results in social media are shown immediately, while the patient's still on the table, instead of months later, when the patient has recovered and the real results can be seen. Patients should check out the doctor's website, make sure they are certified in plastic surgery (or whatever specialty they are seeking), and go to a few consultations. While it can be a helpful part of the puzzle, I wouldn't choose a doctor based entirely on social media.

## HOW MUCH OF SOCIAL MEDIA CONVERSATION ABOUT THE BEAUTY INDUSTRY IS RELIABLE?

**Charles Thorne:** Very little.

**Ashley Gordon:** Unfortunately, not much. A recent study from Northwestern looked at 1.8 million posts that contained plastic surgery-related hashtags, and only 17.8 percent of those came from board-certified plastic surgeons. In my opinion, the percentage of reliable information is probably even less, as many of the plastic surgeons who post the most are more interested in their own celebrity than in educating patients on plastic surgery. I've seen some of their accounts, and it's truly an embarrassment to our specialty.

**Marta Rendon:** It will always depend on the source of the message and the platform used to emit the message. In today's world, everybody should be aware of the perils of misinformation on social media, especially in an industry where marketing can often mislead a patient or consumer into believing that they can reach unobtainable results.

**Adam Rubinstein:** Social media is a great way to search for information and resources about beauty and cosmetic surgery. Some of what you'll find is truthful and very helpful, while other things might be bald-faced lies and deceptions. Just like everything else in life, you have to be careful. The quality of the source is important. That's one of the main reasons I started @plasticsurgerytruths on Instagram and YouTube. Sometimes people have a hard time deciphering what's real and what's not. With @plasticsurgerytruths, I try to clear the muddy waters with good, accurate, and reliable information.

**Clyde Ishii:** The upside of social media is that it's making plastic surgery more mainstream. Most of the posts are harmless. However, anyone can post anything, and there's no filter, so misinformation is very possible. The other issue is that many posts are made by people who are not properly trained to do plastic surgery. It is well known that many lay people pose as plastic surgeons and offer plastic surgery, usually at bargain prices.

**Tracy Pfeifer:** Depends on which social media we are talking about. Any social media that relies on on-the-table results to get their message across is inherently unreliable. On-the-table surgical results do not represent what the long-term, more permanent results will look like and are therefore deceptive. Immediate filler results are more reliable but are also deceptive because of the swelling, which will resolve.

**Armando Soto:** This is very difficult to answer because I really think that as it pertains to our field, all social media must be viewed through the lens provided by a careful understanding of the post creator's overall character as a physician and human being. There are some among us who are excellent marketers, but average physicians, or worse. And some who, quite frankly, are simply entertainers, but whom I would not trust with the care of a loved one. The best among us will demonstrate a healthy balance between marketing themselves and having the appropriate respect for their patients.

"An article was published in *Aesthetic Surgery Journal* showing that only 18% of people using the hashtag #PlasticSurgery were board-certified plastic surgeons. It is a really scary space in social media. Someone can have 2 million followers and have never completed any residency training."
Sheila Nazarian

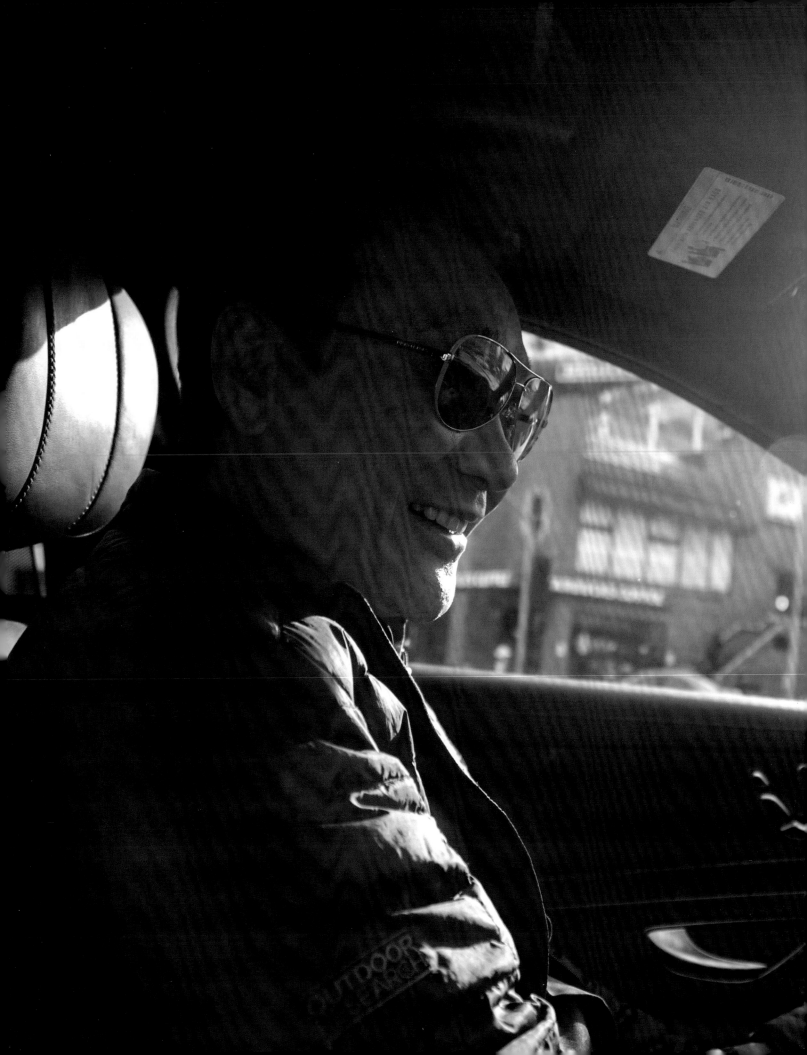

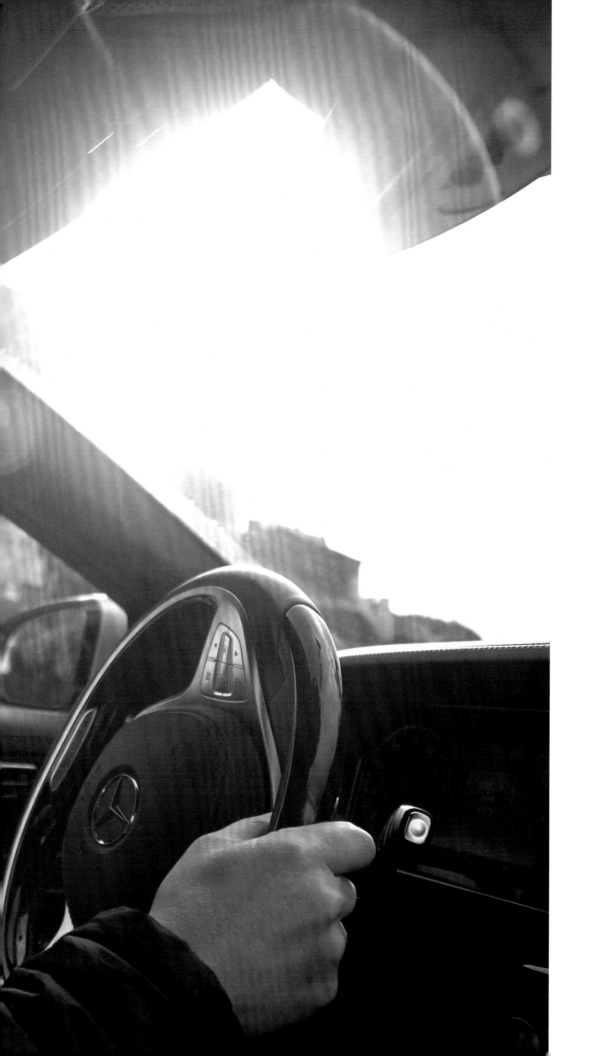

DR. CHARLES S. LEE

IF CHARLES LEE COULD CHANGE one thing about the world, he would make everyone realize that our looks are only part of who we are, that our character is what defines us. Yes, he's a plastic surgeon, in Beverly Hills. And yes, he strongly recommends that anyone interested in a cosmetic procedure first do some serious inner work. Those who think deeply before pursuing plastic surgery are always the happiest patients. They have clear motivations, and they are finding balance in a larger sense.

Balance is what cosmetic surgery is all about. "People seek aesthetic procedures when something's out of whack," Charles explains. "They might not even know exactly what needs to be changed, but there's something that's bothering them, and they want a surgeon to make it right. The improvement always comes down to creating better symmetry or balancing the proportions—sometimes a little of both."

Given his bold assertion that patients aren't ready for surgery until they've clearly defined their inner motivations, it's no surprise that Charles believes in authenticity—authenticity in his relationships with his patients as well as authenticity in the aesthetic he achieves for them.

OUR LOOKS ARE ONLY PART OF WHO WE ARE; OUR CHARACTER IS WHAT DEFINES US.

He believes in a series of consultations with real conversations wherein patients talk about what they think they want, and he helps them determine how to achieve the desired aesthetic. Sometimes patients ask for one procedure when they need something altogether different. Beauty can be a challenging concept for people to articulate; but most people know it when they see it, and Charles's job is to bring them along the path of discovery.

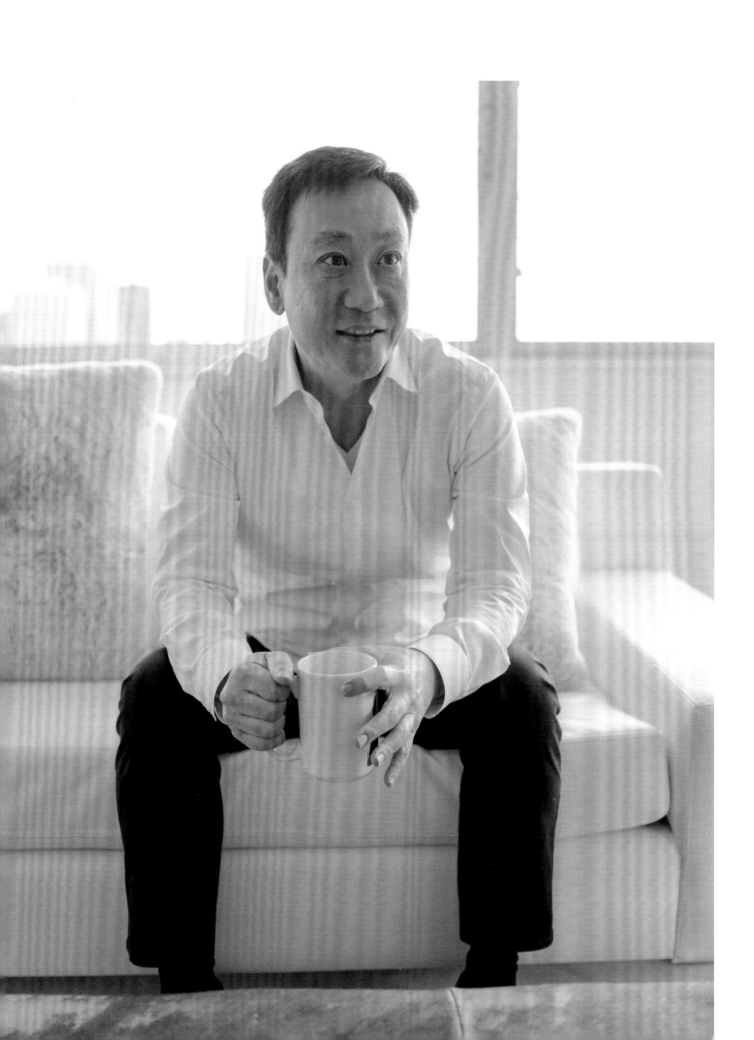

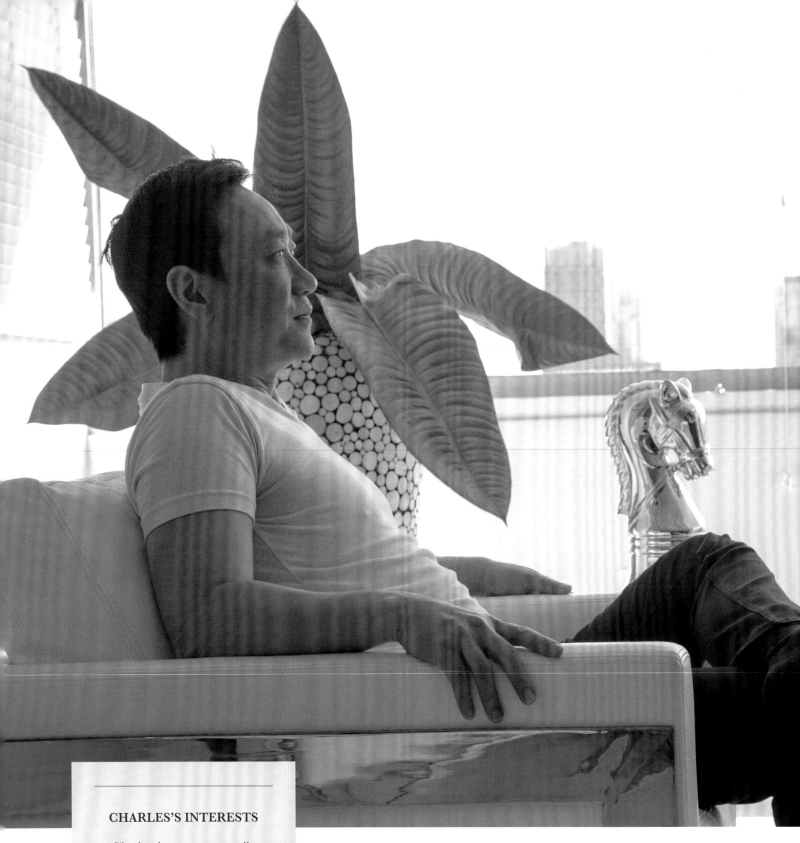

## CHARLES'S INTERESTS

Charles does not necessarily consider himself a conventional artist or a collector, yet he has an honest appreciation for art.

"In the field of medicine, cosmetic surgery is the closest thing to art that you can get," he explains.

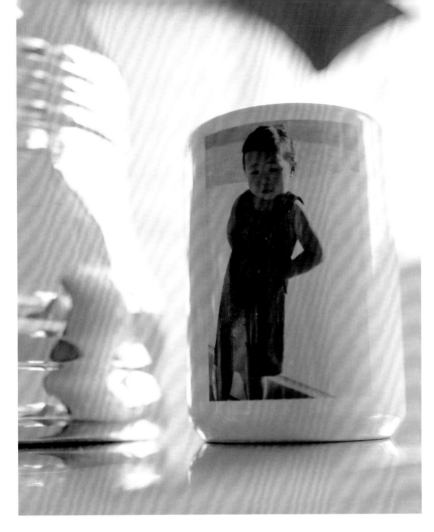

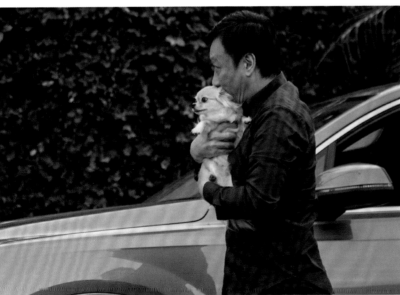

CHARLES SEES HIS FAIR SHARE of celebrities, and it's an honor, to be sure. Yet they are a particularly challenging lot, often expecting their doctors to simply act, no questions asked. Charles doesn't work that way. He is happy to help them so long as he can be a true doctor and give them honest feedback. "When you see celebrities who have had far too many cosmetic procedures and it's clear that they have psychological problems," he explains, "no one has been their doctor, no one has said 'no' to them. Everyone deserves a medical professional who will look out for their best interest."

Celebrity or not, all of Charles's patients appreciate his passion for problem solving. No two surgeries are ever exactly alike because no two people or objectives are ever the same. He may know 95 percent of the tissues and bone structures he will encounter before a surgery, but until he begins operating, there is always an element of mystery. That element is where Charles shines. He likens performing a rhinoplasty to creating a sculpture: "You have it all planned out and you account for as many variables as you can, yet you don't know the exact firmness of the clay until you begin working with it. That's where experience and artistry really come into play."

"When something or someone is interesting enough to make you stop and think and look a little longer—that's beauty."
Charles Lee

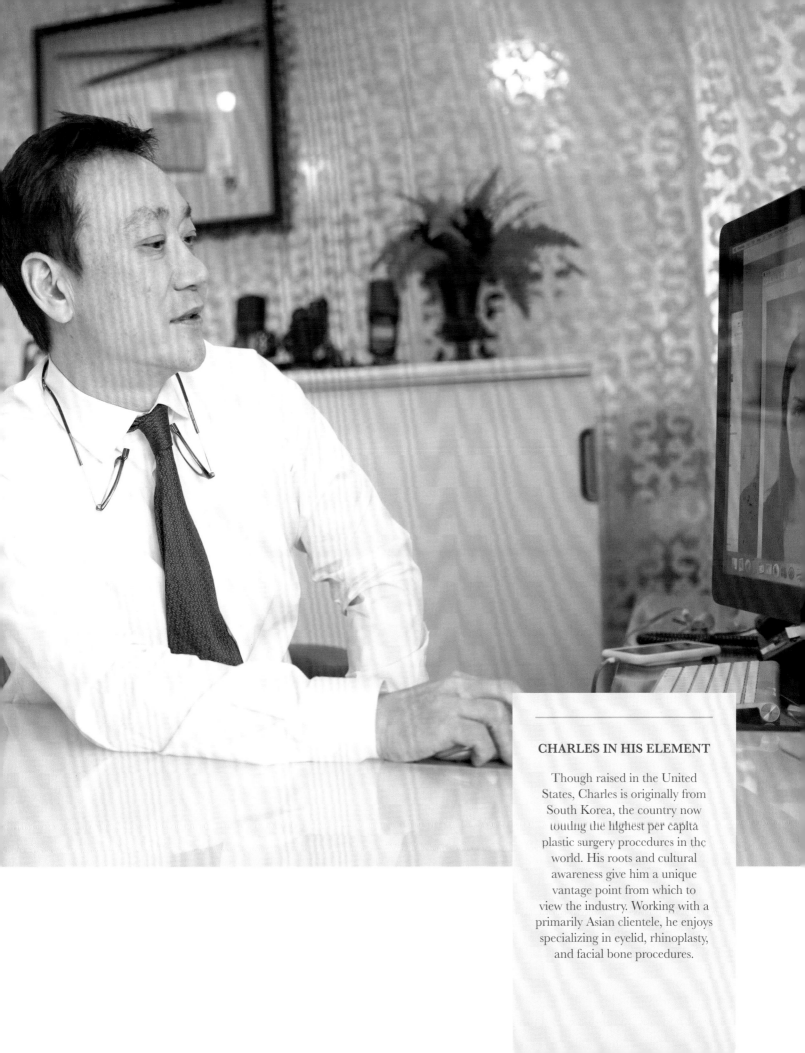

## CHARLES IN HIS ELEMENT

Though raised in the United States, Charles is originally from South Korea, the country now touting the highest per capita plastic surgery procedures in the world. His roots and cultural awareness give him a unique vantage point from which to view the industry. Working with a primarily Asian clientele, he enjoys specializing in eyelid, rhinoplasty, and facial bone procedures.

"Pay a little attention in your 20s, and save yourself headaches in your 40s."
Sheila Nazarian

SKIN

## WHAT ARE THE BEST PROACTIVE MEASURES TO ENSURE A LIFETIME OF GORGEOUS SKIN?

**Clyde Ishii:** Avoid repeated and prolonged sun exposure, ensure proper and diligent use of sunscreen, avoid cigarette smoke, maintain a healthy diet rich in antioxidant foods, and make hydration a priority.

**Robyn Siperstein-Paul:** My top five proactive measures are sunscreen, Retin-A, Botox®, Sculptra®, and photofacials. Sun damage accounts for a majority of skin aging in most people. Protect yourself every morning when you wake up, and reapply. Retin-A has proven in many studies to increase collagen growth, thicken the skin, and remove the outer layer of dead skin for a healthy, beautiful glow. Start at an early age, and apply every night. Botox calms the muscles that cause wrinkles. If you start early, those wrinkles will never have a chance to form. Every year we lose volume in our faces. Using Sculptra® to help rebuild some of that lost volume will help prevent the sagging that eventually occurs. Photofacials have been shown in studies to build collagen and erase the signs of photo-aging, such as red and brown spots.

**Ashley Gordon:** Sunscreen, topical retinoids, and yearly BBL (broad-based light) treatments.

## IS TANNING SAFER THAN BEING IN THE SUN?

**Marta Rendon:** No! Sun exposure is not healthy, as it increases your risk of photodamage and ultimately skin cancers. Tanning is just a delayed response to skin injury from the sun.

## WHAT IS ULTHERAPY®, AND WHO IS IT RIGHT FOR?

**Clyde Ishii:** It is a noninvasive device that uses ultrasound energy to tighten skin at the neck, submental area, and forehead. It also is used to improve wrinkles at the chest. Patients should be informed that the degree of skin tightening and wrinkle reduction may vary from one individual to another. It is indicated only for patients with mild to moderate skin laxity. Patients with greater degrees of skin laxity need surgical correction.

**Sheila Nazarian:** I think it is a good maintenance procedure after a facelift.

## BENEFITS AND DRAWBACKS OF VARIOUS LASER AND LIGHT TREATMENTS.

**Robyn Siperstein-Paul:** There are amazing benefits with light treatments such as Intense Pulsed Light (IPL) or BroadBand Light (BBL) in that they are proven to actually increase the synthesis of collagen while removing brown and red spots on the surface of the skin. The only drawback to this procedure is if you have a recent tan from sun exposure, which makes it difficult for the light to differentiate your tan from your brown spots. This can result in unintended consequences, especially if the treatment is administered by an inexperienced provider or technician at a high setting, as it can remove the tan and cause blistering and pigmentation problems. It is also important to tell your provider if you have any history of cold sores, as light is a known trigger to an outbreak, and you may need to pre-treat with oral medication. Our office has amazing results with both photofacials and laser resurfacing with our Sciton Er:YAG, which is safer than the older CO2 resurfacing. We have many patients who look 10 years younger after their treatments, as we remove all of their wrinkles and start with fresh, new skin.

## HOW CAN RADIOFREQUENCY POSSIBLY DO ANY GOOD?

**Sheila Nazarian:** It is my go-to tightening modality. I have external radiofrequency, radiofrequency with microneedling, and minimally invasive radiofrequency devices, depending on the patient and the aesthetic needs.

**Clyde Ishii:** Radiofrequency devices work by heating the skin's collagen to shrink the skin. For all such noninvasive devices, the degree of skin tightening may vary from patient to patient. Patients with mild to moderate skin laxity may be candidates for this modality. Surgical correction is indicated for those with greater degrees of skin laxity.

SKIN

"Today, aging gracefully includes seeking a little help looking fresh as time and gravity march on."
Adam Rubinstein

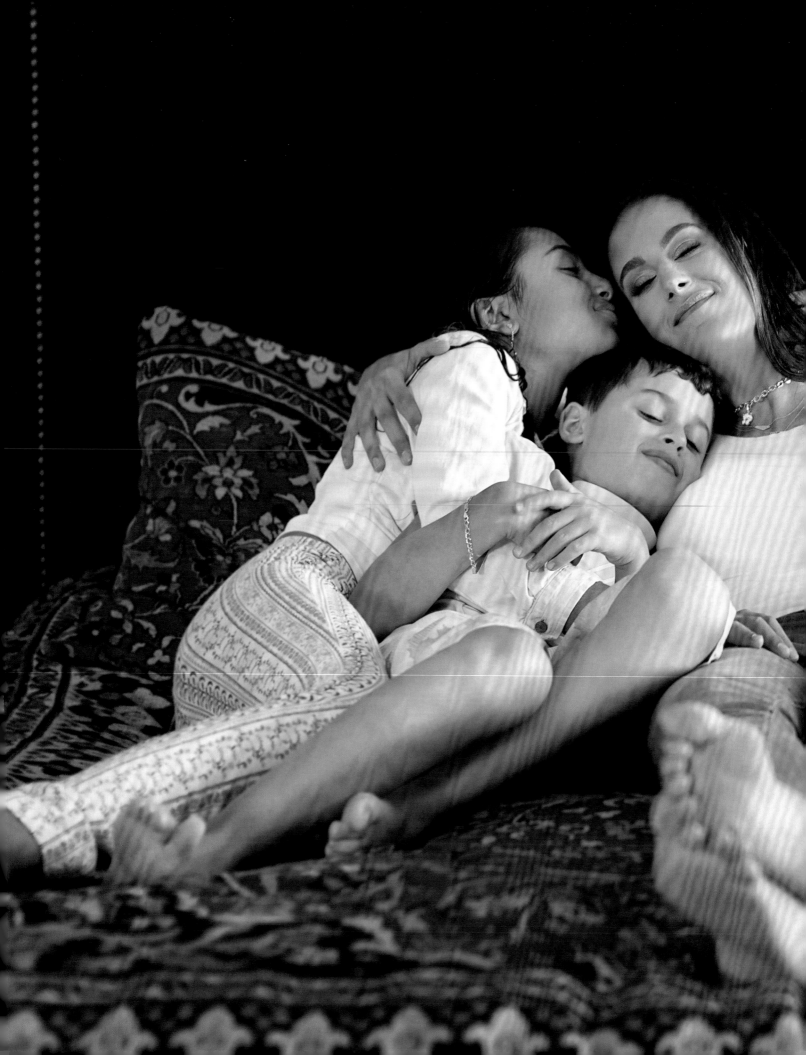

DR. SHEILA NAZARIAN

**M**OST OF SHEILA NAZARIAN'S patients are models, actresses, or moms. Sheila just so happens to have experience with all of these professions, and she's acutely aware of the demands they place on the mind, body, and soul. In the entertainment industry, she was shocked to meet so many people who felt that all they had in the world was their face. If she could change the world, she would empower people everywhere to enjoy their youth while planning for the future, setting themselves up for a new success rather than lamenting the passing of time. "A 40-something model shouldn't be surprised when her career begins to change," she explains.

> 10 PERCENT UNDERDONE IS INFINITELY BETTER THAN 10 PERCENT OVERDONE.

As a surgeon, Sheila certainly has the ability to bestow the fountain of youth on all who seek it; yet she appreciates that this is not in the patient's best interest. Rather than surgically altering every square inch of someone's face or body—which inevitably yields a "fake" look—she much prefers to utilize her skills to help people age gracefully or subtly alter their appearance to become the best version of themselves.

Sheila firmly believes that 10 percent underdone is infinitely better than 10 percent overdone. She fills slowly and carefully to ensure an authentic look every time. "Natural never goes out of style," she says. Sheila has developed her entire practice on this principle, and when new patients come to her "over-filled," she asks them to come back once they've dissolved a bit because she wants them to have the full effect of the aesthetic she develops.

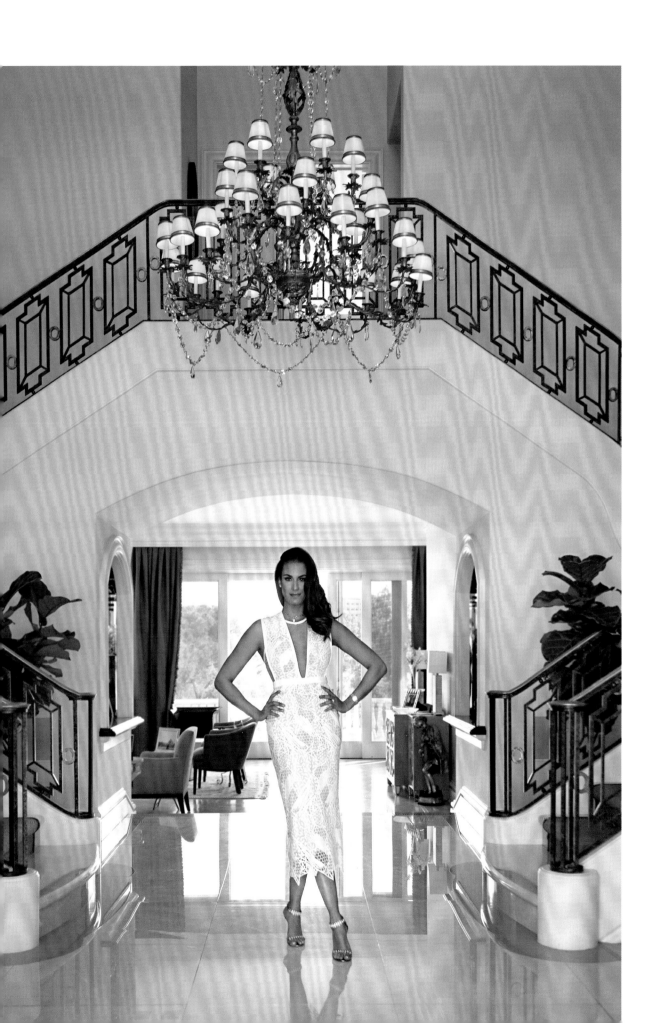

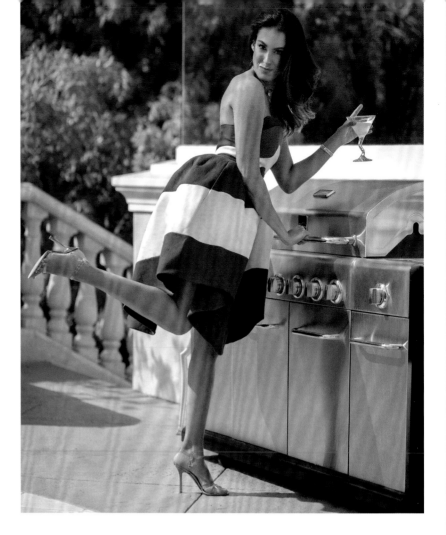

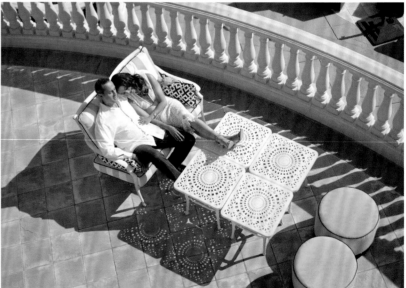

"SOMETIMES PEOPLE in their 50s wake up, look in the mirror, and are suddenly shocked at what they see—and they panic a bit," Sheila explains. "This always surprises me because we actually age the most from our 20s to our 30s." She strongly advises preventative treatments from an early age as a complement, of course, to sun protection and the use of medical-grade skincare products. Sheila is a cosmetic surgeon who loves to operate and give people dramatic results; yet she has surrounded herself with a staff of specialists who perform a full range of noninvasive procedures.

The composition of her practice speaks to her sincere desire to act in the patient's best interest. She believes in making small enhancements to great effect, when possible, rather than simply operating on anyone who inquires. "It's easy for a specialized doctor to tell every patient they're a good candidate for the procedure," she says. "If you want an honest opinion, you have to find a doctor you trust who offers a wide array of surgical and noninvasive procedures. That's how you get the best results."

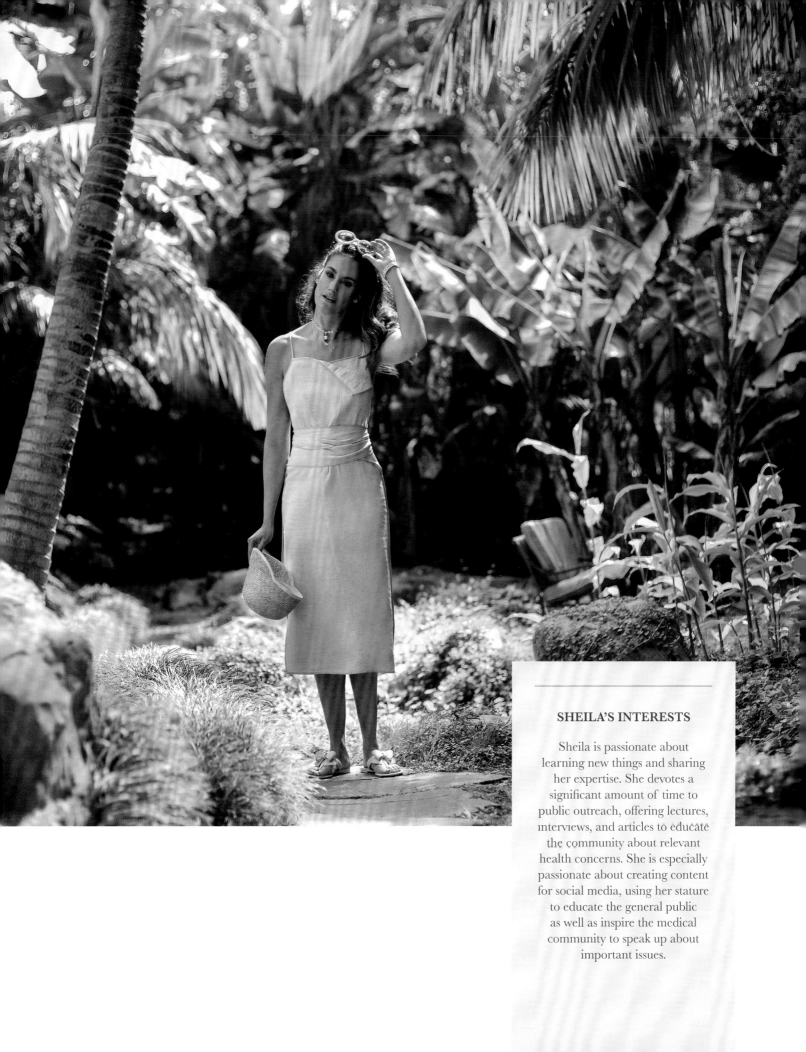

## SHEILA'S INTERESTS

Sheila is passionate about learning new things and sharing her expertise. She devotes a significant amount of time to public outreach, offering lectures, interviews, and articles to educate the community about relevant health concerns. She is especially passionate about creating content for social media, using her stature to educate the general public as well as inspire the medical community to speak up about important issues.

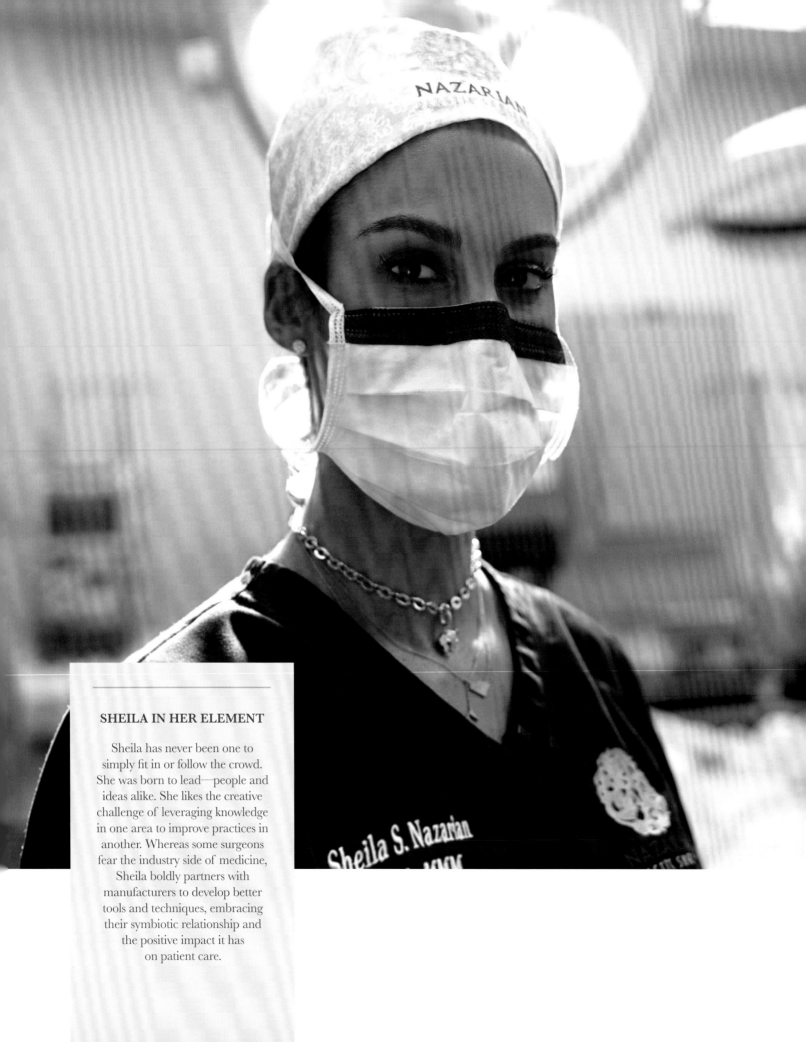

## SHEILA IN HER ELEMENT

Sheila has never been one to simply fit in or follow the crowd. She was born to lead—people and ideas alike. She likes the creative challenge of leveraging knowledge in one area to improve practices in another. Whereas some surgeons fear the industry side of medicine, Sheila boldly partners with manufacturers to develop better tools and techniques, embracing their symbiotic relationship and the positive impact it has on patient care.

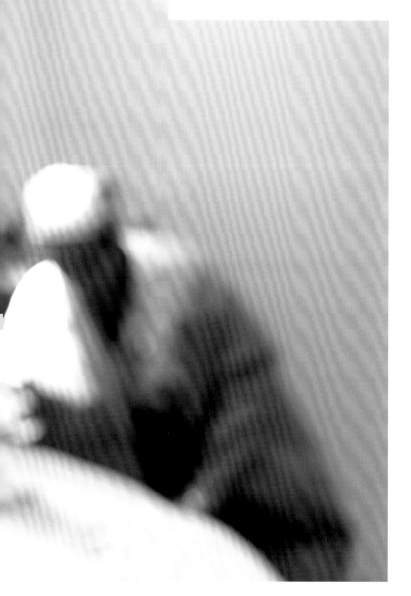

"You don't want to look like anyone else; you want to look like the best version of you."
Sheila Nazarian

"I love to see multigenerational family members together and analyze their faces—what a fascinating study of the commonalities in skin, volume, and bone structure, and how they change over time."
Ashley Gordon

FACE

## WHAT ARE THE BENEFITS OF SURGICAL VERSUS NONINVASIVE FACE PROCEDURES?

**Anna Petropoulos:** We can accomplish a lot with noninvasive procedures. This is where I always begin, because in most cases, I can achieve amazing, natural-looking results—gently, safely, painlessly. Even if a patient chooses the surgical route, the surgery always needs to be followed by annual noninvasive procedures to maintain the aesthetic and protect the patient's investment.

**Richard Warren:** Surgical and nonsurgical procedures each have their own advantages, disadvantages, and indications. Often they are complementary, with a patient getting the most benefit with some of each. Generally nonsurgical procedures are less involved than surgery; they are walk in/walk out procedures, and no anesthetic is required. After the procedure, there is usually little or no recovery time, side effects are fewer, and risks should be minimal. Surgical procedures are the reverse, with much more commitment required by the patient along with the acceptance of more significant side effects. That said, some nonsurgical procedures can do things that surgery cannot, such

as filling fine lines and paralyzing specific muscles. Similarly, surgery can make transformative changes with long-lasting and often permanent results that cannot be achieved any other way.

**Ashley Gordon:** Surgery is still the best at repositioning facial soft tissues with significant vertical descent, causing deep nasolabial folds, jowls, and marionette lines. Fillers can act as a bridge by elevating soft tissues that have minimal to moderate descent. With regard to the facial rejuvenation, we need to look at the position of soft tissues, volume, and skin texture/quality. You can do the best facelift in the world in terms of lifting soft tissues, but if the skin looks like leather, the patient won't really look better or younger. Noninvasive options, like BBL, laser treatments, toxins, PRP, and medical-grade skincare products are integral in our fight against aging. We can't think of surgery and noninvasive as either/or, but rather as complementary.

## WHAT FACE PROCEDURE DELIVERS THE MOST LASTING RESULTS?

**Clyde Ishii:** This has been debated for some time, and the answer is still not clear. Most

plastic surgeons believe that lifting just the facial skin (skin lift) is not very good, as there will be tension on the suture lines resulting in wider scars. Many surgeons today utilize the deeper fascia (SMAS—superficial musculo-aponeurotic system) layer to do the lifting but vary the modification of the SMAS according to the patient's facial shape. For patients with a wide midface, the SMAS is tightened, thereby lifting the attached fat. This procedure is called SMAS plication, or SMASectomy. Patients with a narrower midface may benefit from a procedure called high SMAS, or extended SMAS. The SMAS layer is elevated and recruits attached tissue to the cheekbone area, thereby increasing the transverse dimension of the midface area. Transplantation of fat (fat grafting) is usually added to the facelift procedure to combat facial volume loss that occurs with aging.

**Richard Warren:** In the world of facelift surgery, there is much debate about the best way to do the procedure. Today, most experienced surgeons agree that the skin is a covering layer that is not designed to hold up heavy facial features. Therefore, repositioning the deeper tissues of the face—mostly fat and some muscle—is the key to facelift longevity. There is disagreement over exactly how the deep tissues should be handled. I am in the camp of surgeons who believe that, for most patients, a dissection and repositioning of the deep facial tissues (called the SMAS layer) will provide the most longest-lasting result. I also think that fat grafting for the volume-depleted face is a major adjunctive procedure with the advantage of permanence.

**Robyn Siperstein-Paul:** Using Bellafill® in combination with laser resurfacing creates amazing, long-lasting results. While Bellafill® has been shown to last the duration of a five-year study, I have seen it last even longer in my patients.

## WHAT ARE YOUR THOUGHTS ON COSMETIC EAR SURGERY?

**Jim Grotting:** Patients with prominent ears usually seek the counsel of a plastic surgeon prior to first grade. The summer before first grade is the ideal time for surgical correction to prevent the bullying that can occur among small children when a child looks different. People who live with prominent ears spend their lives feeling self-conscious about them and often try to disguise them with ear-hiding hairstyles. Parents who tell their children that they need

to be strong and suffer the teasing are doing them harm, as this deformity can be safely and easily fixed. No child would elect to have ears that stick out when they could be normal after a straightforward surgical procedure.

## HOW DO YOU ENSURE GREAT RESULTS WITH A RHINOPLASTY?

**Jim Grotting:** Probably in no other area of cosmetic surgery is patient education more important than in rhinoplasty. There are so many variables that influence the outcome, that even among the best nose surgeons in the world, we have about a 15 to 20 percent revision rate. It is purely and simply an inexact science. Nevertheless, if the goal is creating the best nasal shape and function for a particular patient with limitations of baseline anatomy, the chances of great results rise considerably. Thick skin, weak cartilages, deformed internal anatomy, and other facial features all influence the result. We simply cannot give every patient the nose that they might pick out of a beauty magazine. That is all part of a well-done preoperative consultation. That being said, rhinoplasty is one of the most powerful cosmetic procedures we perform and can have a remarkably positive effect on self image.

## WHAT DOES A FACELIFT FEEL LIKE AND HOW INTENSE IS THE RECOVERY?

**Charles Thorne:** Some say "it was nothing." Others say "that was no picnic." In either case they are totally recovered in three weeks.

**Richard Warren:** A facelift can be done under sedation or a general anesthetic. In the immediate post-operative phase, there is usually not much pain because the local anesthetic we use is normally still effective for the first few hours after surgery. As the local anesthetic wears off, there will be pain in the cheeks and neck that normally resolves over the first 48 hours. Because of the repositioning of deep tissue, there will be a feeling of tightness in the deep layers of the neck and cheek. Finally, the skin of the cheeks in front of the ear will be quite numb. The patient's first week involves low-key activity, remaining under close observation, and having dressings changed and stitches removed on a preplanned schedule. Most people look swollen and somewhat bruised for about two to three weeks and are usually willing to be seen in public by about three weeks after surgery.

**Armando Soto:** Facelift surgery is actually very well tolerated and associated with minimal discomfort. Most patients say the face feels puffy and tight for a few days.

## WHAT'S THE AVERAGE COST OF A FACELIFT IN THE U.S.?

**Richard Warren:** According to statistics from the American Society for Aesthetic Plastic Surgery, the average surgeon fee for a two- to three-hour facelift is $7,503. However, this figure is misleading. Additional fees will include anesthesia (which may involve another doctor), the fee for the facility in which the procedure is done, and possibly a fee for an overnight stay. Those fees will bump the total up to around $10,000 to $12,000. In addition, if a surgeon does a more complex procedure involving such things as deep tissue dissection, fat grafting or resurfacing, the duration will be longer—perhaps three to four hours. That will bump the fee to the $15,000 to $20,000 range. Lastly, there is considerable variation depending on the geography and the reputation of a surgeon. The highest facelift fees will be found with the most experienced surgeons in the largest cities where fees above $30,000 are common.

## LESSER-KNOWN FACTS ABOUT PERMANENT MAKE-UP PROCEDURES?

**Robyn Siperstein-Paul:** Permanent makeup is not like a body tattoo because it uses FDA-approved pigments that are subject to more rigorous testing and oversight than conventional tattoo ink. If the permanent makeup pigments are not top-quality, the brow colors can fade to peach or pink. Generally when the service is offered at a deeply discounted price, the equipment and pigments used are from countries where the approval process is not so rigorous. Most people are told that microblading is not a tattoo, which is false, as any color implanted into the skin is a tattoo. Microblading is a technique that is done by hand and not with a machine, which is not the best option for every client. The same optimal result—a natural hair-stroked, fluffy brow—can be achieved with a machine as well, with potentially longer-lasting results and less trauma to the skin. As for permanent makeup as eyeliner, not everyone is a candidate. If the patient is too old, with wrinkles or bumps on the lids, the outcome will likely be poor. A skilled and experienced permanent makeup artist will be able to assess a patient's skin to determine the best treatment options.

"Performing cosmetic surgery is like renovating a house. We work with an existing structure and try to improve it. We are not creating a new one."
Richard Warren

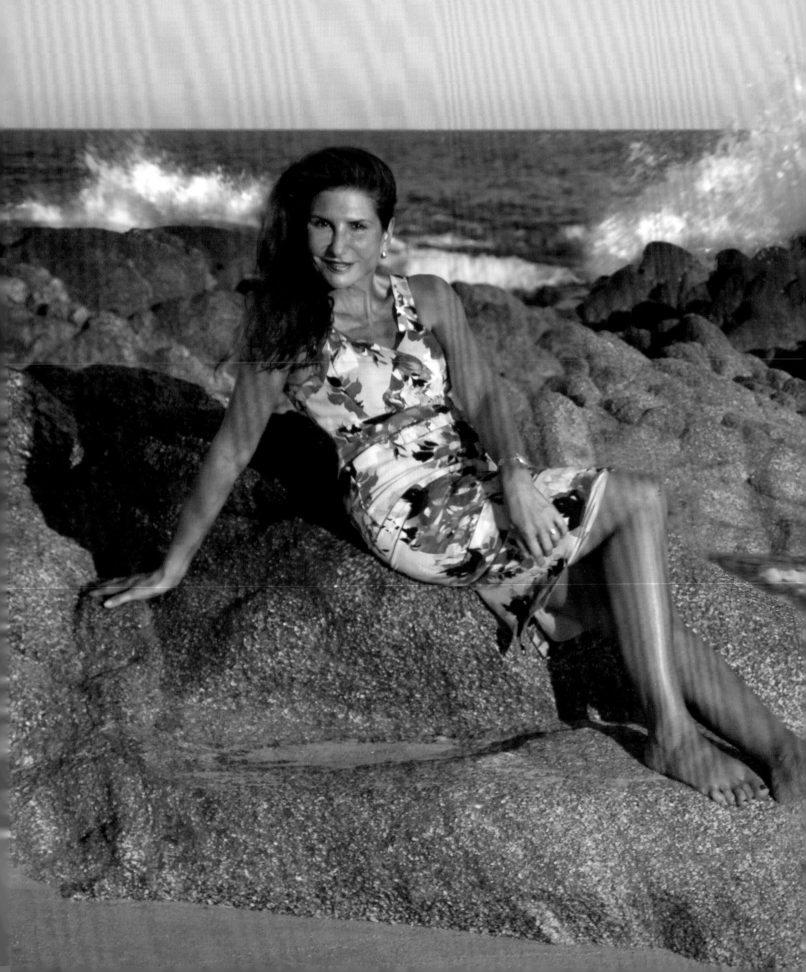

DR. ANNA PETROPOULOS

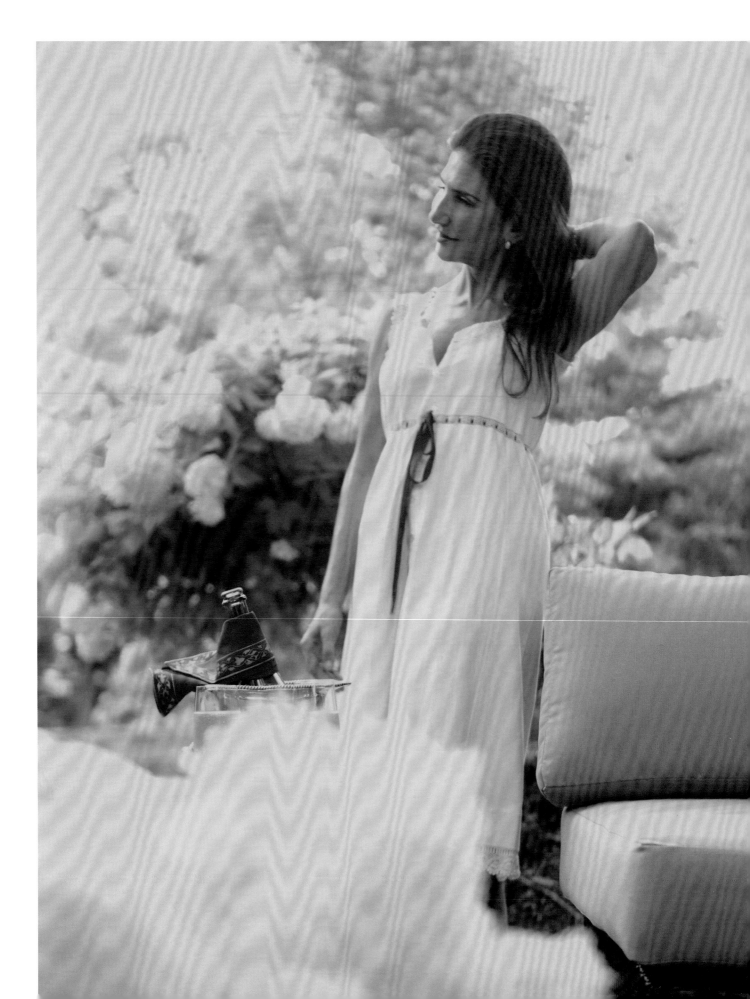

ANNA PETROPOULOS CREDITS her well-honed aesthetic style to her mother and aunt, whose beauty, femininity, and fashion sense are matched only by the gracious manner in which they carry themselves. Of course, Anna's sense of style and passion for achieving visual harmony were also profoundly influenced by her international upbringing—she lived in Africa, Germany, France, and California, regularly vacationing in Greece to visit extended family. One of her fondest childhood memories is studying the classical sculptures of Athens with her parents and marveling at their artistry and timeless beauty. The daughter of surgeons and professors who regularly socialized with other medical professionals, academicians, and diplomats, Anna was blessed to be surrounded by impeccable role models and to have early exposure to a wide world of meaningful career paths.

During college, Anna earned her pilot's license, received a medical research grant from NASA, and was on track to become an astronaut. However, shortly after starting her aesthetics rotation in residency at Harvard, Anna knew she had found her calling. Throughout her career, she has subscribed wholeheartedly to the

A TRADITIONAL FACELIFT MAY DELIVER FAST RESULTS, THOUGH IT'S FAR FROM A ONE-STOP SOLUTION.

philosophy of timeless classical beauty and the power of noninvasive procedures to maintain a natural, youthful look. Surgery plays an impressively small role in this surgeon's practice because she can almost always achieve the results her patients desire using noninvasive techniques. She has more than a dozen different machines in her office and regularly upgrades and updates her technology to ensure that she can offer the safest, most effective treatments possible. While a traditional facelift may deliver fast results, Anna is quick to point out that this popular option is far from a one-stop solution, as regular noninvasive maintenance is still required to protect the patient's investment in their facelift or other surgical procedure. Thoughtfully, gently, and gradually, Anna restores patients to more youthful versions of themselves. When new patients walk through her doors, she doesn't need photographs from their glory days, she simply closely looks at their face and eyes and pictures in her mind what they looked like a few years back—and in some cases, a few decades back.

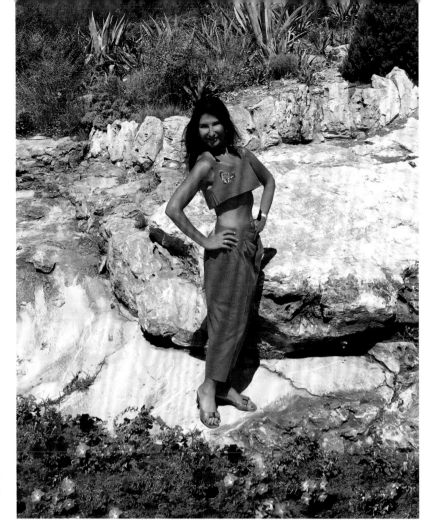

ANNA ADVOCATES proactively preserving a youthful appearance by addressing the main ways in which we age. Regular fillers stave off the development of dynamic and static wrinkles. Annual skin tightening minimizes the expected annual quarter-inch drop of our jaw line and the drooping of our eyelids. Using medical-grade skincare products, including those that utilize stem cell technology, encourages youthful skin texture. A variety of noninvasive techniques can gently reposition tissue to address any inherent volume loss or shift. Taking these steps toward a more beautiful appearance, Anna believes, creates more self-confidence, which, in turn, leads to healthier relationships, better professional performance, and ultimately greater happiness. "This is not a vain profession," she says, "we are helping people by enhancing the way they look, feel, and live."

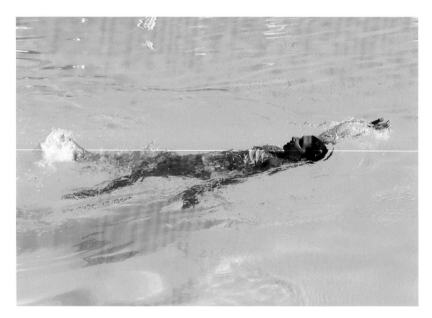

The vast majority of Anna's patients have been coming to her for nearly two decades, so she has formed close relationships, even friendships with them. Her quiet demeanor and the peaceful vibe of her office create an atmosphere where meaningful conversations and transformations are possible. She considers her profession not merely medical or cosmetic but also deeply spiritual. She's like the center of the wheel and her patients are the spokes—through conversations about the ups and downs of life, they are able to anonymously help one another. Fostering internal peace, enhancing physical beauty, and bringing a sense of goodness into her patients' lives motivates and inspires Anna each and every day.

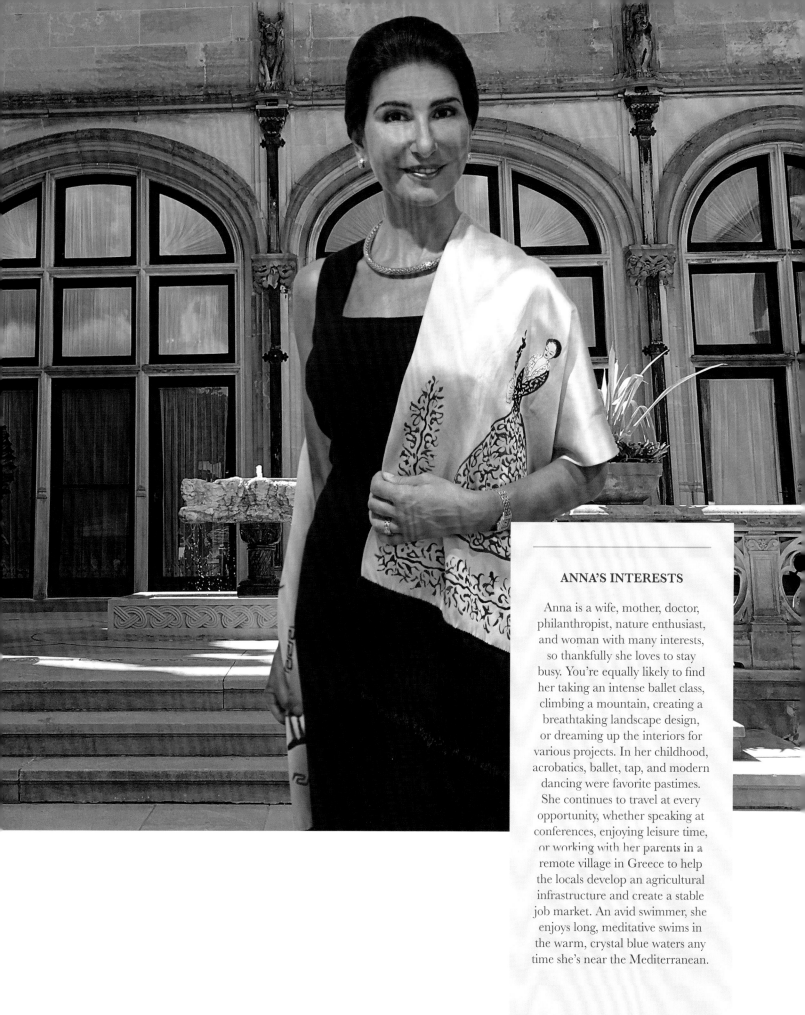

## ANNA'S INTERESTS

Anna is a wife, mother, doctor, philanthropist, nature enthusiast, and woman with many interests, so thankfully she loves to stay busy. You're equally likely to find her taking an intense ballet class, climbing a mountain, creating a breathtaking landscape design, or dreaming up the interiors for various projects. In her childhood, acrobatics, ballet, tap, and modern dancing were favorite pastimes. She continues to travel at every opportunity, whether speaking at conferences, enjoying leisure time, or working with her parents in a remote village in Greece to help the locals develop an agricultural infrastructure and create a stable job market. An avid swimmer, she enjoys long, meditative swims in the warm, crystal blue waters any time she's near the Mediterranean.

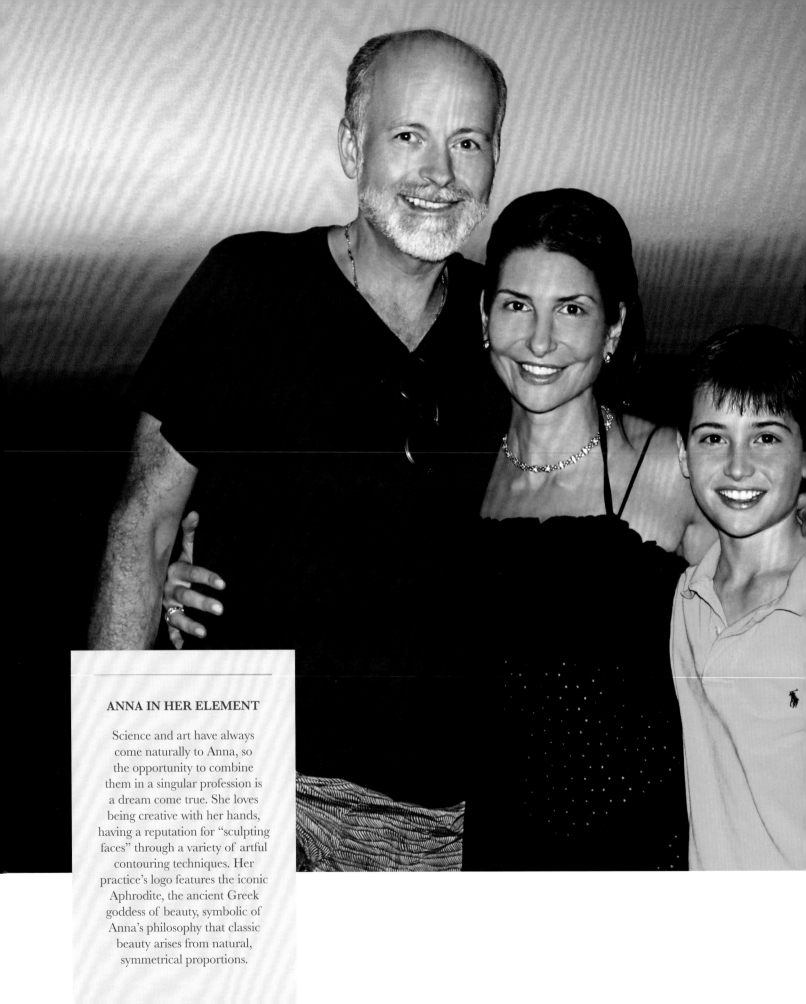

## ANNA IN HER ELEMENT

Science and art have always come naturally to Anna, so the opportunity to combine them in a singular profession is a dream come true. She loves being creative with her hands, having a reputation for "sculpting faces" through a variety of artful contouring techniques. Her practice's logo features the iconic Aphrodite, the ancient Greek goddess of beauty, symbolic of Anna's philosophy that classic beauty arises from natural, symmetrical proportions.

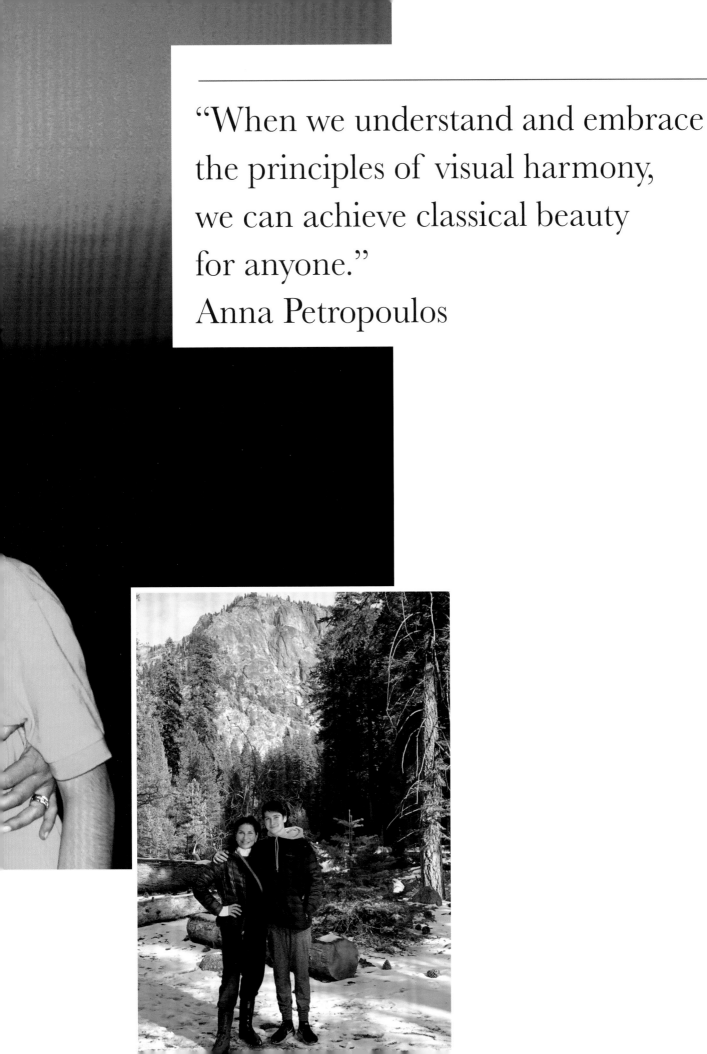

"When we understand and embrace the principles of visual harmony, we can achieve classical beauty for anyone."
Anna Petropoulos

"Breast augmentation is associated with a very high satisfaction quotient compared to other cosmetic surgical procedures."
Clyde Ishii

BREASTS

## HOW BIG IS TOO BIG?

**Clyde Ishii:** Most patients undergoing breast augmentation desire to look more proportional and fit better in clothes. The best results occur when there is adequate soft tissue (breast and fat) to cover the implant. What is too big for one patient may be fine for another patient. A very large implant in a normal-sized patient will often result in breasts that look unnatural because the implant size has outstripped the overlying soft tissue cover. An experienced surgeon will make recommendations regarding implant size based on a dimensional analysis of the patient's chest: tissue thickness, breast width, intermammary distance, skin tightness, etc. Patients who want to look natural must trust that the surgeon will deliver the result based on the preoperative examination.

**Ashley Gordon:** One size does not fit all, so what may be too big on one person is perfect on another. It's all about balance, proportion, patient desire, and tissue quality. I use tissue-based planning to avoid implants that are too big for the soft tissue envelope, because I want a result that's not only going to look great at one year, but also at 10 years and beyond.

**Richard Warren:** Breast size is an extremely complicated and emotionally charged subject. Enlarging breasts by inserting breast implants under the breast is really a very simple concept. However, it does involve creating a large space under the breast and then stretching the overlying tissue to accommodate a foreign object, which inevitably causes some damage to the surrounding tissue. The end point depends on the size of the woman's frame, the elasticity of her tissues, and the size of her existing breasts. A history of pregnancy or the plans for future pregnancy also play into the equation. There are also long-term consequences which must be considered because the larger the implant, the more distortion there may be, and the more likelihood there is that some sort of revision procedure will be necessary in the future. All of these surgical concerns are weighed against the patient's wishes, and therein lies a common problem: the expectations of the patient. Although it may technically be feasible to insert excessively large implants that a patient has requested, the risks of tissue damage and bad long-term sequelae may make this an unreasonable prospect for the surgeon.

**Armando Soto:** I usually believe that beauty is in the eye of the beholder, but on the other hand, I am uncomfortable doing anything to a patient that I believe is going to compromise her safety either in the short term or later in life. If I am being asked for a breast size that will negatively affect my patient's lifestyle or employment options, or increase the likelihood that she will need many more operations in the future because of the choice, I will discuss this with her very carefully.

## HOW LONG DO AUGMENTED BREASTS REALLY LAST, AND WHEN IS IT TIME TO GET THEM REDONE?

**Richard Warren:** There is no "best before date" with modern breast implants. They can safely be left in place until some event comes along to make replacement necessary. For most women for whom there is nothing wrong, it is reasonable to undergo regular surveillance with physical examination and medical imaging, such as a mammogram or breast MRI, after 10 years. Some of the indications for breast implant replacement are saline implant deflation, ruptured silicone gel implant (usually seen on mammogram or MRI), capsular contracture (scar around the implant), implant malposition, and very commonly the desire for implant size change (going bigger or smaller). Some older women simply want to have their old breast implants removed. Also, patients who later in life may have a mastopexy (breast uplift) after pregnancy and who have older implants in place may choose to replace these implants while they are under the anesthetic for the mastopexy.

**Clyde Ishii:** Augmented breasts may look great for many years if they are not affected by pregnancies, capsular contractures around the implants, or implant rupture. Patients undergoing breast augmentation with saline-filled implants do not need to get them checked or replaced unless the implant deflates. The FDA recommends that patients with silicone gel-filled implants get an MRI to rule out implant rupture three years after implantation and then every two years thereafter. Most patients do not abide by this recommendation because they find it too onerous. Therefore, many surgeons recommend at 10 years that these patients either get an MRI or replace the implants.

**Ashley Gordon:** Longevity depends on so many factors: age of the patient, skin quality, whether they've had children and/or breastfed, and size and type of implant, just to name a few. We no longer tell patients that they need to replace their implants every 10 years. Each patient is unique, so I assess each patient's specific situation, and we determine together when it's time for a breast revision and implant exchange. If they are unhappy with size, shape, and/or position, we discuss the various options and focus on the procedure that will minimize the need for future surgery. My surgical plan is always an attempt to break the revision cycle. Thankfully we now have products like dermal matrices and meshes that we use to support the soft tissues, minimize complications, and extend our surgical results.

## WHAT KIND OF PSYCHOTHERAPY IS OR SHOULD BE REQUIRED TO ACCOMPANY SUCH A MAJOR EVENT AS BREAST SURGERY?

**Clyde Ishii:** A good candidate for breast augmentation should not need any psychotherapy. Such a candidate is an emotionally stable adult who has put some thought into getting this procedure rather than doing it on a whim, is undergoing the procedure for herself and not for someone else, has realistic expectations, and is in good health. I would be very hesitant to operate on a patient who is undergoing psychotherapy in preparation for surgery.

**Ashley Gordon:** Psychotherapy isn't required; rather, a good plastic surgeon should invest quality time with patients during their consultations. Besides a thorough exam, I like to spend time just getting to know them, hearing about their motivations, seeing their wish pictures, and reviewing before and after pictures of similar patients. Great plastic surgeons usually have high emotional intelligence, so this helps with identifying any red flags.

**Richard Warren:** I don't think the average, level-headed woman who requests breast implant surgery needs to be referred to a psychologist for psychotherapy. However, the patient who has psychological issues should not proceed with surgery until her mental state has been investigated and dealt with. As with any cosmetic procedure, patients shouldn't proceed with breast augmentation unless they are mentally and emotionally stable.

## WHO IS A GOOD CANDIDATE FOR A BREAST LIFT?

**Jim Grotting:** Breast ptosis, or drooping of the breast, occurs with large heavy breasts, postpartum atrophy, or loss of support and stretching of the skin following pregnancy and lactation, and sometimes due to deformity during development in adolescence. All of these patients benefit by lifting with or without the support of an implant or even fat grafting to the breast. A major mistake in aesthetic surgery of the breast is to try to treat drooping of the breast with large implants to take up the loose skin. This inevitably leads to a large, low breast that makes fitting of clothing and swimsuits difficult and almost always requires the eventual reoperation with smaller implants and a breast lift.

## WHAT DOES RECOVERY FEEL LIKE, REALLY, AND IS IT WORTH THE PAIN?

**Ashley Gordon:** I hear patients every day say, "It was so much easier than I thought it would be." Always trying to improve the patient experience, I adopted an enhanced recovery protocol where medications that decrease inflammation, muscle spasm, and nerve-type pain are utilized in place of narcotics. Most patients are back to their lives in just a few days and report minimal discomfort after breast surgery. This also prevents all of the side effects associated with narcotics, like constipation, itching, and potential dependence.

**Armando Soto:** It depends on the details of the surgery being performed and on the personality of the surgeon and the patient, too! I think that a lot of the pain experienced by patients after elective surgery can be related to anxiety and how well it is managed, both by the surgeon and the staff, and the patient and her friends and family. In my practice, even the most painful breast operation is usually described as some pressure and moderate discomfort by the vast majority of patients. I cannot recall a single patient who would not say that the recovery wasn't worth the pain.

**Clyde Ishii:** The recovery varies according to how the procedure is conducted, the anatomic level of the implant (subglandular vs. submuscular), the size of the implant relative to the skin laxity, and the use of long-acting local anesthetics. A very thin nulliparous patient undergoing a submuscular breast augmentation with relatively large implants (going up more than one cup size) with no long-acting local anesthetic will experience a fairly significant amount of postoperative pain and tightness for about one week or so. She will not feel "normal" for at least two to three weeks. On the other end of the spectrum is a patient who has had one or more children, has a fair amount of skin laxity, and is undergoing a subglandular augmentation with small/moderate-sized implants. This patient will have minimal discomfort, and her recovery will be much faster. Most patients who have undergone the procedure feel it was very worth it, even considering the postoperative discomfort. The use of local anesthesia pain pumps or long-acting local anesthetics has really helped minimize postoperative pain. Breast augmentation is associated with a very high satisfaction quotient compared to other cosmetic surgical procedures.

## HOW MUCH DOES BREAST SURGERY COST?

**Richard Warren:** Regarding cost, according to statistics from the American Society for Aesthetic Plastic Surgery, the average surgeon's fee for a 1–2 hour breast augmentation is $3,990. However, this figure is misleading. Additional fees include anesthesia (which may involve another doctor), the cost to purchase the breast implants themselves, and the fee for the facility in which the procedure is done. Those fees will bump the total up to between $7,000 and $10,000, depending on the type of implants used, the geographical location, and the experience of the surgeon.

**Armando Soto:** The costs of breast surgery will depend on the details of the procedure, who the surgeon is, and where it is being done. The least expensive breast procedure in my practice would cost approximately $6,000, and the most I have charged for a complex, multistage revision or reconstruction of a complicated problem was $24,000.

## HOW CAN YOU TELL IF THEY'RE NATURAL OR SURGICALLY PERFECTED?

**Ashley Gordon:** If they look perfect, they probably aren't natural.

**Clyde Ishii:** Many times it is difficult to tell if breasts have been augmented, especially if the implants are on the smaller side. Sometimes the scar is a giveaway. Augmented breasts in thin patients with implants above the chest wall muscles often appear unnatural because there is insufficient soft tissue cover. Patients with submuscular implants may have an animation deformity—when the pectoralis muscles are flexed the breasts move. However, this takes a trained eye to detect.

**Armando Soto:** I would know a good job was done if I saw the patient in a bikini on the beach and found myself admiring the outcome as a natural look rather than something surgically achieved.

**Jim Grotting:** With a well-done breast augmentation, one should wonder whether the breasts are real or surgically enhanced. Giveaways as to the presence of an implant are a very rounded upper pole where one can almost see the upper edge of the implant, which often becomes worse if there is hardening or capsular contracture around the implant. Also, when the implant ripples or wrinkles in a patient with scant breast tissue, one can detect the presence of an implant. Usually petite, slender women who have had large implants placed appear a bit disharmonious, and it is easier to detect the breast implant.

"With a well-done breast augmentation, one should wonder whether the breasts are real or surgically enhanced."
Jim Grotting

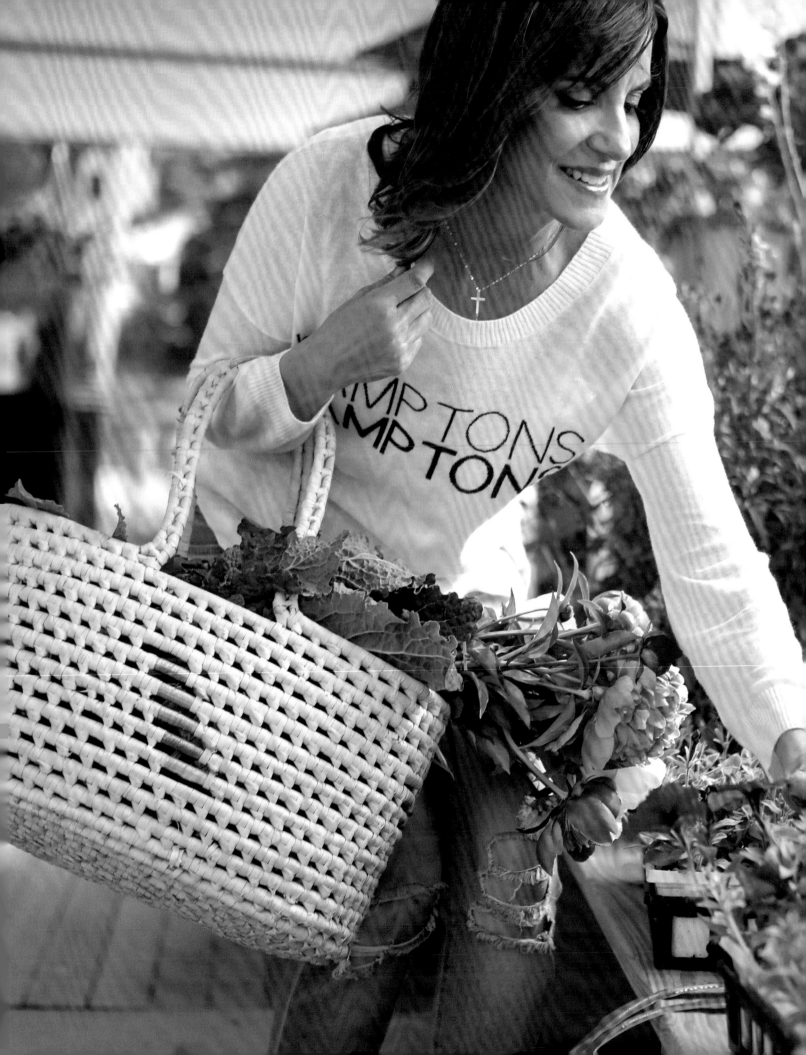

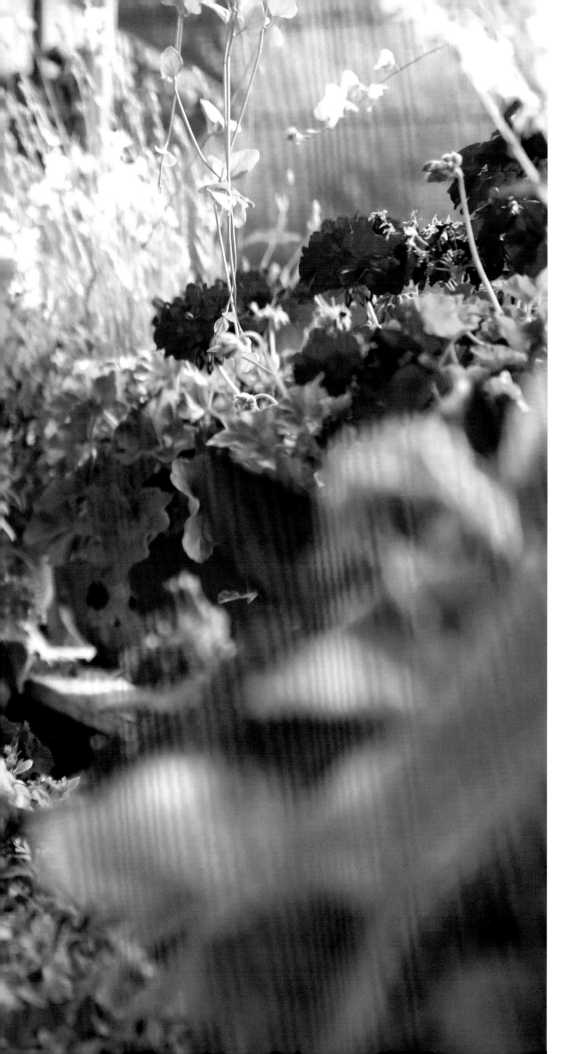

DR. TRACY PFEIFER

# T

RACY PFEIFER BELIEVES THAT WE ARE NOT here to have a frivolous life. Rather, we are here for the purpose of elevating the lives of those around us using our unique talents. Her unique talents? A confident mind, well-trained hands, and the eyes of an artist. A true Sagittarius, she is the type of person who loves to learn—anything. Whether in the realm of aesthetic surgery, history, design, or something totally obscure, newfound knowledge is a joy to Tracy. The more she learns about a topic, the more she appreciates and enjoys it. This zest for personal growth and development serves her well as she helps patients refine their appearance.

> WE ARE HERE FOR THE PURPOSE OF ELEVATING THE LIVES OF THOSE AROUND US USING OUR UNIQUE TALENTS.

Like most aesthetic surgeons, Tracy references the golden proportions; however, she is quick to note that the patient's lens is most important, even if it doesn't necessarily align with her personal ideal of beauty. The patient needs to feel great about the results. Tracy is adept at talking people through the basics of beauty theory—how the perfect breasts on one person might be altogether wrong on another—and partnering with them to discover the look they truly want and the best way to achieve it.

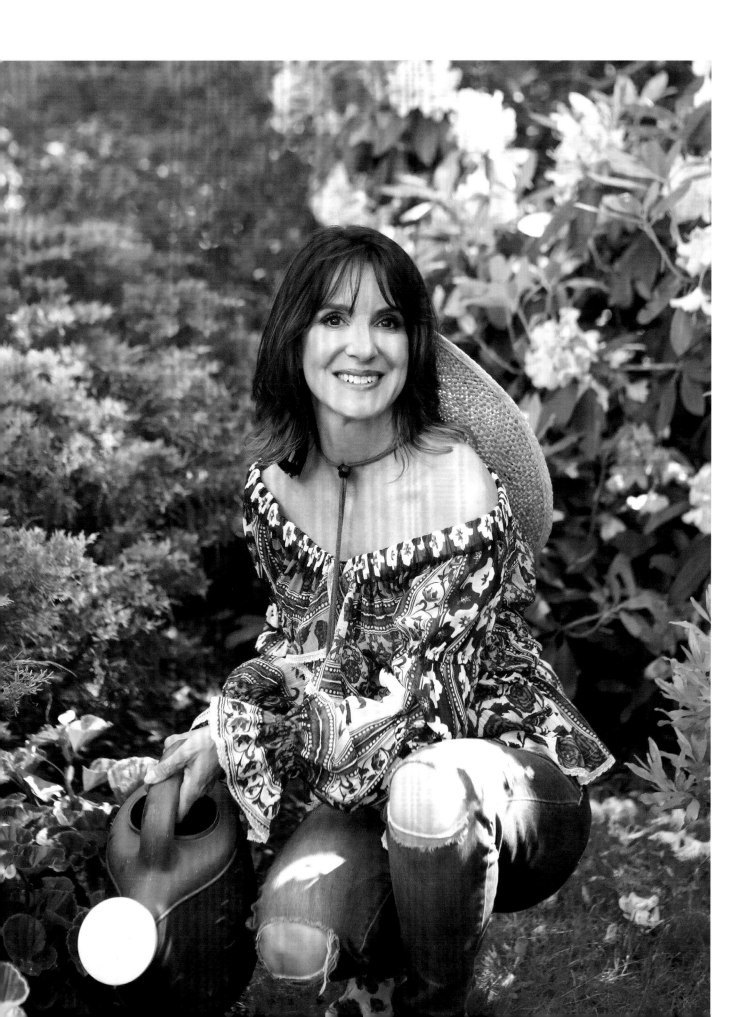

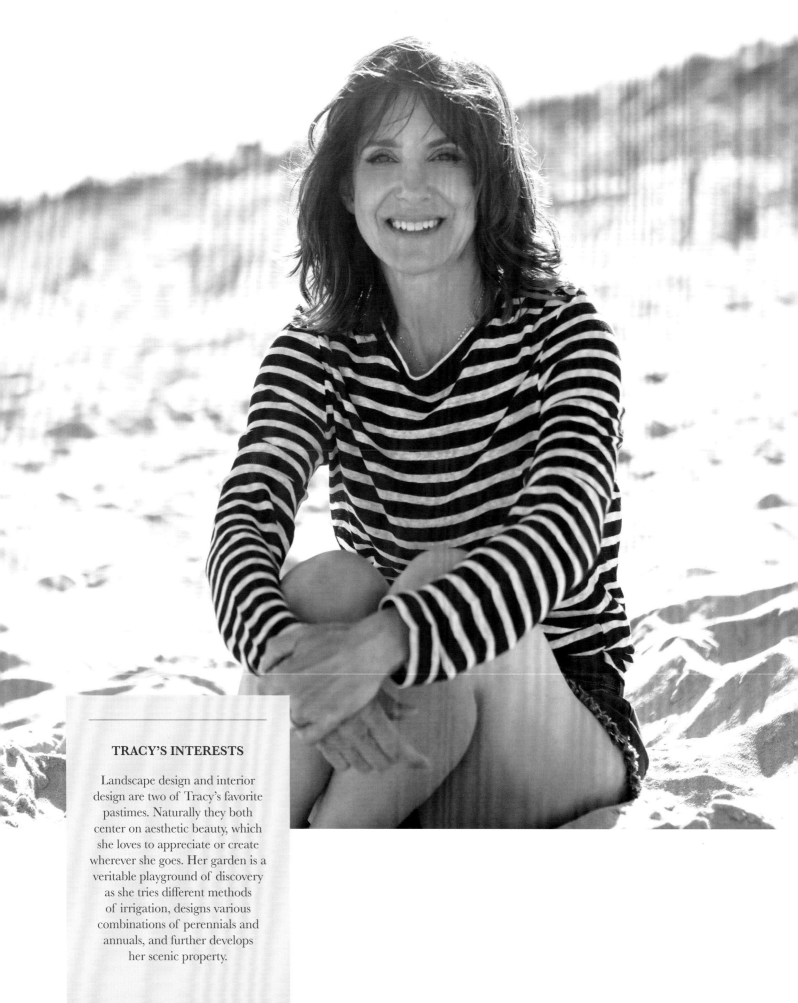

## TRACY'S INTERESTS

Landscape design and interior design are two of Tracy's favorite pastimes. Naturally they both center on aesthetic beauty, which she loves to appreciate or create wherever she goes. Her garden is a veritable playground of discovery as she tries different methods of irrigation, designs various combinations of perennials and annuals, and further develops her scenic property.

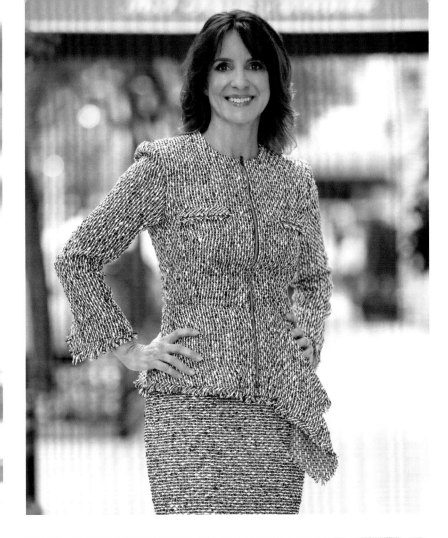

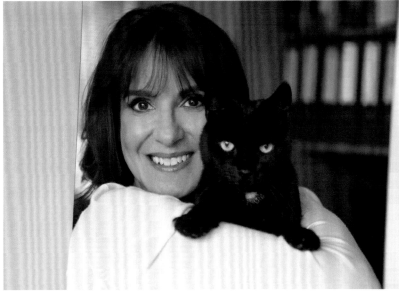

"AESTHETIC SURGERY ISN'T copy and paste," she explains. "There are many possible solutions to every challenge. Good surgeons take great care to determine the best approach for each patient." By planning each surgery and respecting principles of beauty, she ensures the natural look that patients desire. New patients usually reveal "looking natural" as their first concern. As soon as they learn the basic statistics on how many people undergo aesthetic surgery, they realize that many of the "naturally beautiful" people they admire have had their beauty enhanced by a surgeon.

A seasoned professional, Tracy can sometimes spot surgical procedures when she is out and about—the silhouette of an implant that's a little too large on a slender person, or fat injections that achieve a fullness not normally found in certain ethnicities, for instance. But by and large, when the work is properly performed and proportions are respected, the only people who should be able to tell if someone has work done are the patient's family and closest friends. To the world, well-performed surgical procedures have the potential to be imperceptible.

"Beauty is the golden proportion, which applies to everyone and everything—from classic architecture to seashells."
Tracy Pfeifer

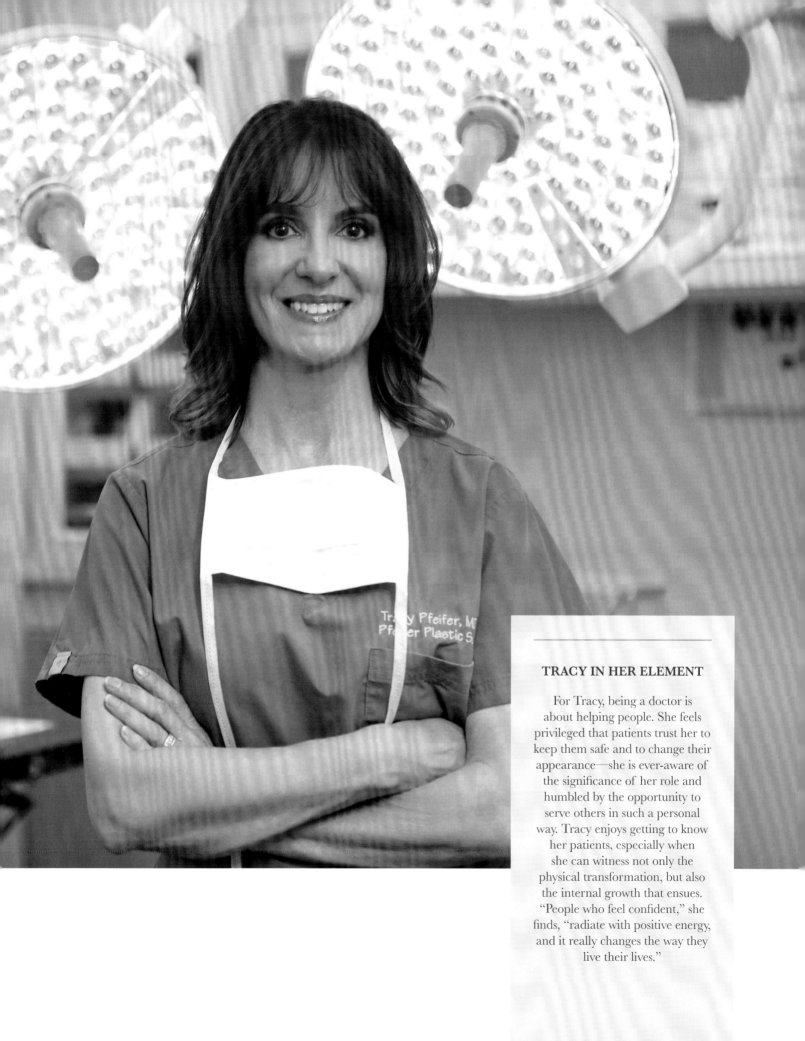

### TRACY IN HER ELEMENT

For Tracy, being a doctor is about helping people. She feels privileged that patients trust her to keep them safe and to change their appearance—she is ever-aware of the significance of her role and humbled by the opportunity to serve others in such a personal way. Tracy enjoys getting to know her patients, especially when she can witness not only the physical transformation, but also the internal growth that ensues. "People who feel confident," she finds, "radiate with positive energy, and it really changes the way they live their lives."

"In this profession, we see people at their very worst and their very best—patients, as well as those who are supposed to love them unconditionally. It's humbling. My wish is for everyone to know true compassion."
Armando Soto

BODY

## WHAT DOES A TUMMY TUCK ENTAIL?

**Jim Grotting:** A tummy tuck involves the correction of displaced rectus muscles which become unhinged during pregnancy or major weight gain, as well as the removal of excess skin and fat of the lower abdominal wall. The muscle repair is what keeps the abdomen flat. It almost always requires some liposuction of the waist and hip rolls. The removal of the skin will leave a long low scar, but most patients gladly trade the scar for the flat abdominal contour. Women who undergo tummy tucks remark that their clothes fit remarkably better, and that even bowel and bladder function can be improved.

## TELL US ABOUT FAT TRANSFERS. WHERE DOES IT COME FROM, AND WHERE DOES IT GO?

**Clyde Ishii:** Fat grafting or transfers are used to augment areas of fat loss that occurs with aging (temples, cheeks, lips, etc.) or to augment a normal area (breast, buttock). Fat is harvested from a variety of donor sites: abdominal wall, hip roll, flanks, thighs, medial knees, etc.

**Ashley Gordon:** Donor fat can come from almost anywhere, but the most common sites are abdomen and flanks. I personally like donor fat to come from areas that are resistant to diet and exercise, because when I transfer it, I want it to stay. I don't want weight fluctuations to impact my result. The most common recipient sites are the face, the breasts, and the buttocks, but fat can be used anywhere to correct contour issues from trauma, botched surgery, and congenital problems, just to name a few. Fat is also rich in stem cells, so when we perform fat transfer, we not only get the benefit of enhanced volume, but also the regenerative effects of the stem cells on the skin.

**Armando Soto:** Ideally, the fat is coming from an area of relative excess and is being placed in an area the patient would like to see have more fullness and contour.

## IS COOLSCULPTING® A VIABLE OPTION?

**Armando Soto:** It is an excellent option for the right patients. Unfortunately, this is a much smaller group than is seeking improvement. It works best for those with smaller areas of excess fat, good skin tone, and tight muscles.

**Clyde Ishii:** It does work but is usually reserved for selected areas (love handles, lower abdominal wall, submental area). Some patients get better results than others, so all patients must be properly counseled. It is a good option for patients who want to avoid surgery if at all possible.

## IS LIPOSUCTION STILL A THING, OR IS THERE SOMETHING BETTER?

**Clyde Ishii:** According to the 2016 statistics from the American Society for Aesthetic Plastic Surgery, liposuction remains the number one cosmetic surgical procedure in the United States.

**Ashley Gordon:** Liposuction is still the gold standard for permanent fat reduction, but the technology, surgical approach, instrumentation, and techniques have evolved. My focus is never just on fat reduction but rather on re-contouring. How can I balance the patient's shape and proportion? And what does the patient desire? SAFELipo® is my go-to technique because it offers not only fat reduction, but predictable skin contraction and amazing results. I also use High Def liposuction in patients who desire a very athletic look.

**Armando Soto:** Liposuction is an excellent option—and is, in fact, still the gold standard for improving the shape of the body, when muscle tightening and skin removal are not necessary. Modern liposuction often involves ancillary procedures like ThermiTight® or BodyTite.

## HOW MUCH FAT REDUCTION CAN BE ACCOMPLISHED IN ONE SURGERY?

**Armando Soto:** Quite a bit. Most surgeons agree that the limit of safety in one session is about four to five liters of floating fat. This would represent a very large amount of suction—there are very few patients who are simultaneously good candidates for liposuction and who need that much removed. Most people who would need more fat than that removed should probably be having a different operation.

**Ashley Gordon:** Five liters of fat, sometimes more, can be safely suctioned in one sitting, but to get a stellar result, the focus should be on re-contouring, not just fat reduction. If the patient has a pear shape and you significantly reduce just her trunk and not her thighs, she will look out of proportion, and her clothes will not fit properly.

**Clyde Ishii:** Contouring of the abdomen is limited to the abdominal wall. Some patients have a protuberant abdomen, with most of their girth due to intra-abdominal fat and only a minor contribution from fat in the abdominal wall. These patients need to reduce their internal fat load through diet and exercise, as liposuction of the abdominal wall will not make much of a difference. On the other hand, patients with most of their fat in the abdominal wall and whose skin elasticity is good make great candidates for liposuction. Significant improvement is possible in these patients.

BODY

## HOW MUCH DOES LIPOSUCTION RECOVERY HURT?

**Armando Soto:** Liposuction of the abdomen usually feels like you did way too many sit-ups the day before: achy and crampy. Most patients take pain medicine for two to three days.

**Ashley Gordon:** It depends on the area treated and the technique used. In my experience, the arms, inner thighs, and back are the most tender after surgery. Discomfort is easily managed with appropriate post-op pain protocols.

**Clyde Ishii:** There is mild to moderate discomfort associated with liposuction, but the patient recovers fairly fast since the muscle and other deeper structures are not affected.

## HOW PERMANENT ARE THE RESULTS OF LIPOSUCTION?

**Armando Soto:** The results of liposuction are long-lasting since fat is being permanently removed from the areas treated, and humans don't (under normal circumstances) produce more fat cells. This is what leads to the most commonly held myth surrounding liposuction—that having liposuction in one area of your body will result in collecting fat disproportionately in other areas. For example, you will often see reports of women who had liposuction on their abdomen and say that a year later their thighs and butts were huge. They are telling the truth—their butts and thighs are now larger—but the liposuction was not the cause. Sometimes, when you liposuction a patient's abdomen and waist, they find their clothes are loose in these areas and they start to eat more. Then because they now have many fewer fat cells in the abdomen where fat can collect, it collects in the areas where fat cells still exist in abundance: thighs, butt, and arms.

**Ashley Gordon:** With liposuction, the fat cells that are removed are gone forever, so in that sense it's permanent. However, if someone goes on to gain weight, fat cells in other areas of the body will expand.

**Clyde Ishii:** The results are fairly permanent provided that the patient maintains their preoperative diet and exercise regimen. Many patients turn over a new leaf once they achieve the new body contour. These patients feel good about their new physique and rev up their exercise program. On the other hand, there are patients who fall off the wagon, and their results are not so permanent.

## WHAT PROCEDURES DELIVER THE SAFEST, FASTEST RESULTS?

**Armando Soto:** The goal should always be the safest, most beautiful results. If, at the end of your plastic surgery experience, you can say that you were safe and the results were seen quite soon after a minimal recovery, but you look weird, funny, or unattractive, I promise you will not consider it to have been a positive experience. On the other hand, even if your recovery is just a bit longer (but still acceptable), but you feel equally cared for and safe, and your appearance is beautiful and natural, then you (and those who love you) will always feel the decision to have plastic surgery was one of the best you've made.

**Ashley Gordon:** In my hands, SAFELipo® delivers the safest, fastest, and most permanent results.

"People who feel confident radiate with positive energy, and it really changes the way they live their lives."
Tracy Pfeifer

BODY

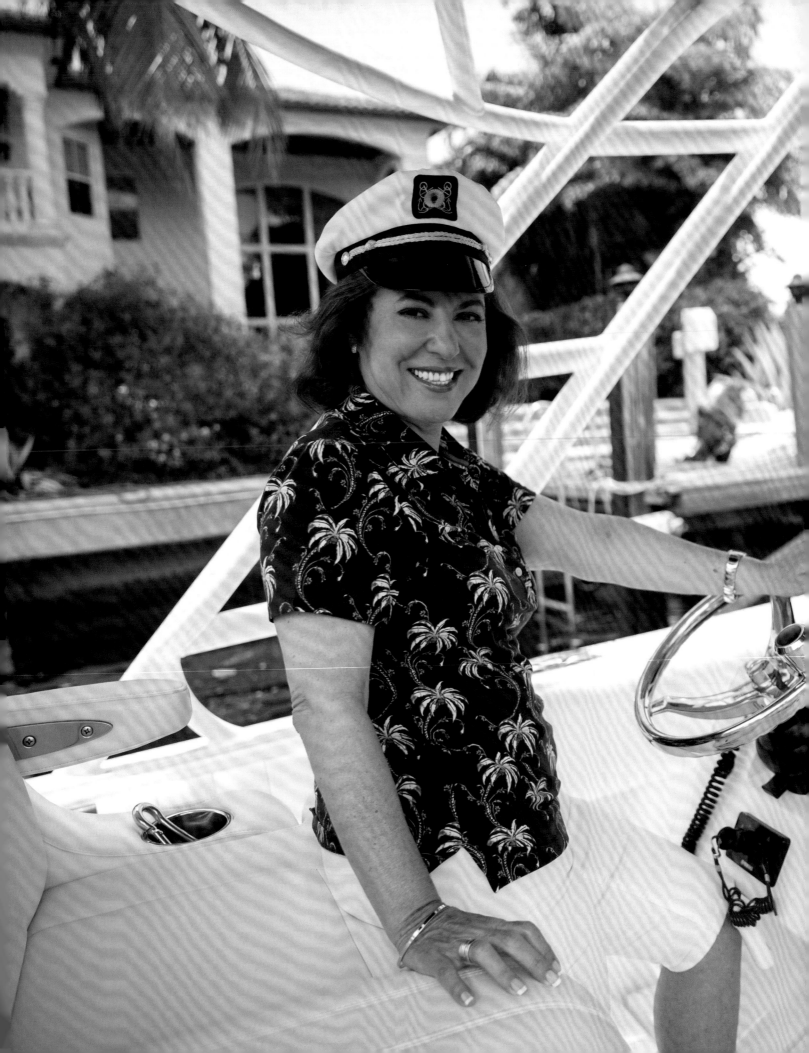

DR. MARTA RENDON

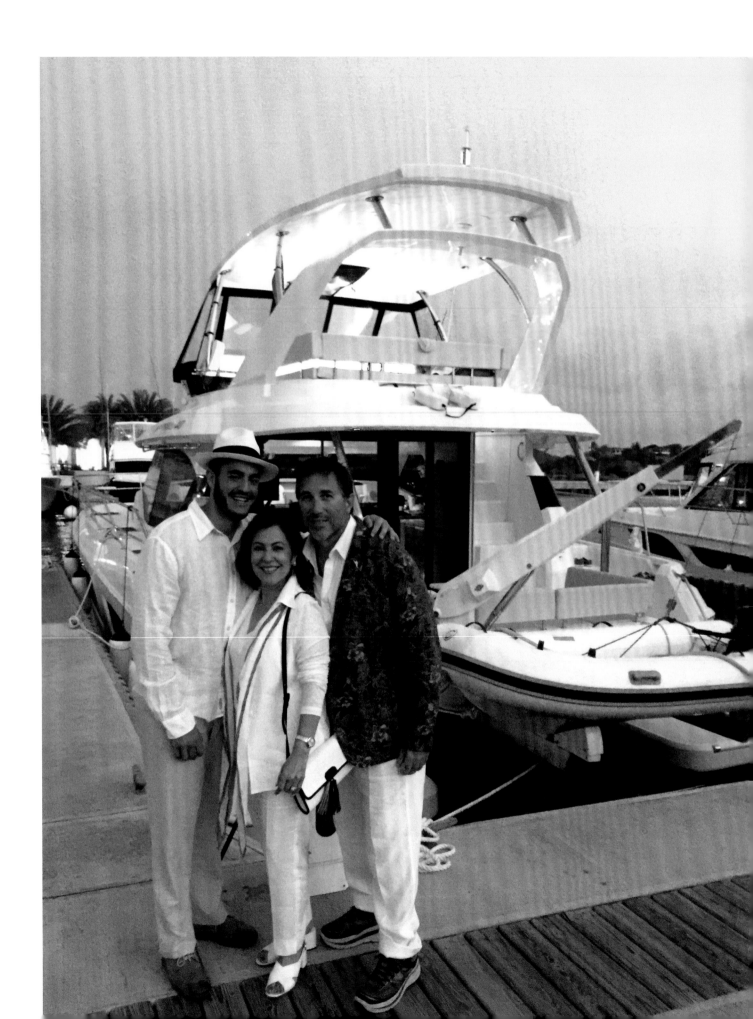

# M

ARTA RENDON IS A DERMATOLOGIST and skin-care researcher known for her big heart, charming laugh, and radiant personality. Although she is board-certified in dermatology and internal medicine, she is more than a physician: She is an artist who helps patients find their inner and outer beauty, and a friend whom her patients trust will provide the best advice.

Using dermatological mediums like fillers, Marta artistically transforms the way shadows flow and light reflects to turn people into better versions of themselves. "When fillers are done really well," she explains, "even your best friends won't be able to tell what you had done; but they'll recognize that you look amazing."

Marta brings an interesting perspective to the aesthetics scene, because she is double-board certified in internal medicine and dermatology. Utilizing her unique blend of specialized knowledge, she has developed a rare talent for diagnosing diseases and conditions far earlier than many would think possible. Colon cancer, ovarian cancer, and diabetes all have subtle internal and external symptoms that, when realized together and treated early, can prove lifesaving. Practicing with such great attention to detail earned her the nickname "Eagle-eye Rendon," which she embraces as the highest compliment. "To do great work in aesthetics," she explains, "you have to have an artistic eye as well as impeccable motor skills. Lots of people have one or the other; having both is what differentiates the masters from everyone else."

> ARTISTICALLY TRANSFORMING THE WAY SHADOWS FLOW AND LIGHT REFLECTS CAN TURN PEOPLE INTO BETTER VERSIONS OF THEMSELVES.

Relationships are important to Marta. She believes in working hard to earn people's trust and keep it. This mantra combined with her intrinsic need to be among the first to know of every technological advance—has led to a number of opportunities to work with major pharmaceutical companies and other manufacturers who know she only supports things that are safe and ethical. She weighs in on the effectiveness of new products and methodologies, throwing herself into her research, never hesitating to speak her mind about her discoveries. When the science backs up the company's findings, she shouts her enthusiasm from the rooftops and is the first to bring the product or method to her patients. When the science is lacking, she speaks just as loudly.

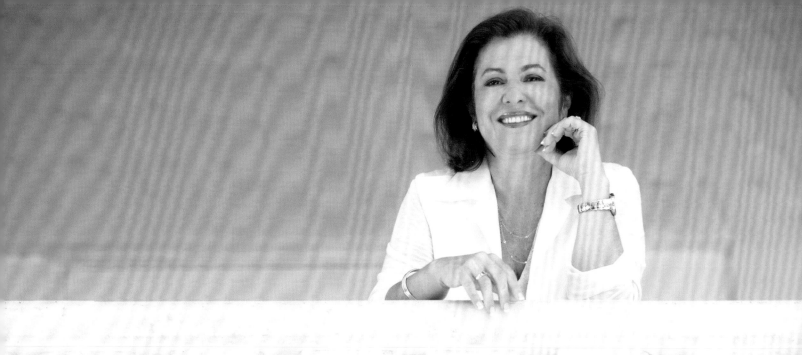
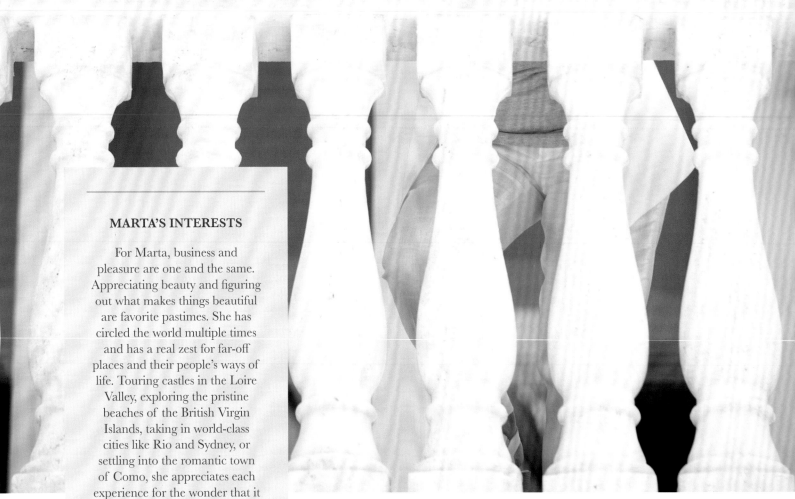

## MARTA'S INTERESTS

For Marta, business and pleasure are one and the same. Appreciating beauty and figuring out what makes things beautiful are favorite pastimes. She has circled the world multiple times and has a real zest for far-off places and their people's ways of life. Touring castles in the Loire Valley, exploring the pristine beaches of the British Virgin Islands, taking in world-class cities like Rio and Sydney, or settling into the romantic town of Como, she appreciates each experience for the wonder that it brings. She'll go anywhere yet is particularly drawn to regions with the blissful combination of rugged mountains meeting vast bodies of water—and of course places with inimitable architectural character and deep historical meaning are always welcome.

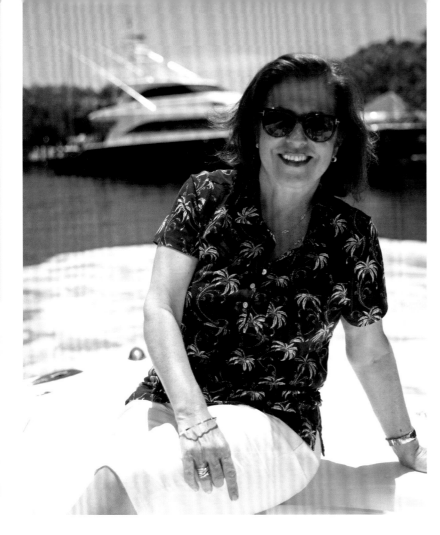

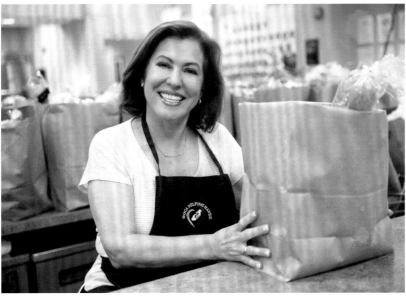

WHILE SOME DOCTORS ARE too polite to offer their opinions on what needs to be altered, Marta is always willing to directly yet diplomatically express her professional recommendations. She begins consultations by handing patients a mirror and asking what they're focused on. Then she asks permission to tell them what she sees and how she can enhance their look. She finds that this technique really opens the lines of communication and that most people are relieved to have the candid observations and advice of an expert. One day, out of the office, she asked a casual acquaintance if she'd ever considered doing anything about a large scar on her face caused by an accident. The woman was initially taken aback and then quickly became excited at the prospect of a solution to something that had burdened her for so long. Those moments when Marta can open up possibilities to effect positive change in people's lives are what keep her pushing forward in the art and science of achieving higher forms of beauty.

Perspectives on beauty vary widely, yet Marta believes that all definitions encompass the principle of harmony. "When you look at something or someone beautiful," she says, "you're overcome with peace, you feel good, and your brain relaxes because your eyes are experiencing what your soul craves: harmony."

"Have aesthetic procedures to make yourself happy. You deserve to smile when you look in the mirror."
Marta Rendon

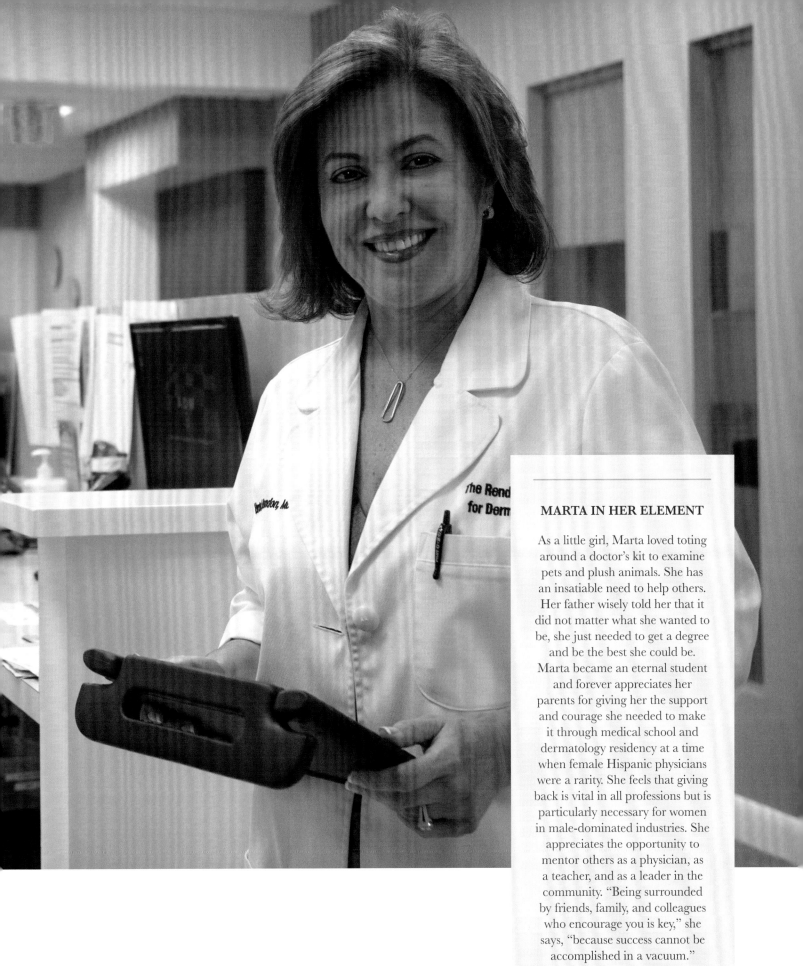

## MARTA IN HER ELEMENT

As a little girl, Marta loved toting around a doctor's kit to examine pets and plush animals. She has an insatiable need to help others. Her father wisely told her that it did not matter what she wanted to be, she just needed to get a degree and be the best she could be. Marta became an eternal student and forever appreciates her parents for giving her the support and courage she needed to make it through medical school and dermatology residency at a time when female Hispanic physicians were a rarity. She feels that giving back is vital in all professions but is particularly necessary for women in male-dominated industries. She appreciates the opportunity to mentor others as a physician, as a teacher, and as a leader in the community. "Being surrounded by friends, family, and colleagues who encourage you is key," she says, "because success cannot be accomplished in a vacuum."

"The oversized butt is a trend, and hopefully one that will go away soon; but the results of surgery don't go away when the trend does."
Ashley Gordon

BUTT

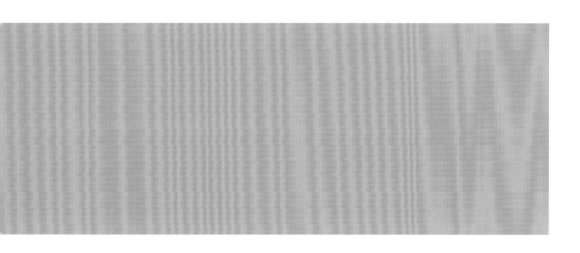

## WHY DO BRAZILIANS USUALLY GET ALL THE CREDIT?

**Ashley Gordon:** Ivo Pitanguy, a pioneering Brazilian plastic surgeon, was the first to describe fat transfer to the buttock; hence the name Brazilian Butt Lift. Unfortunately his technique has been bastardized here in America by the Kardashian effect.

## LET'S TALK TIMELESS VERSUS TRENDY, AND GO.

**Ashley Gordon:** In my opinion, a vast majority of buttock augmentations being performed in the US today are failing patients. The oversized butt is a trend, and hopefully one that will go away soon; but the results of surgery don't go away when the trend does. It won't be as simple as suctioning the fat out, because the skin envelope will be over-stretched, and removal of volume will just result in ptosis or sagginess. Surgeons are going to have to develop lifting procedures to deal with deflated skin envelopes and sagging of buttock tissues due to gravity and the weight of the enlarged butt. This will likely include unsightly scars with increased risk of infection due to their challenging location. As a

specialty, we frequently deal with the negative consequences of oversized implants on breast tissue, so I'm surprised and disappointed that surgeons in our specialty are ignoring these lessons and not applying them to patients requesting oversized buttocks. If patients were truly educated on tissue consequences of high-volume buttock augmentation, many would opt out of the surgery or at least request a more reasonable size.

**Armando Soto:** The current trend, of course, is to have a large, round behind created using your own fat. My strong opinion, and what I strive for in my own patients, is a timeless shape and size that ages well with them, and most women seeking this type of surgery don't understand the difference. Let me explain: The vast majority of women seeking this type of surgery are young—in their 20s or 30s. Their metabolism reflects this youthfulness at the time of surgery. But as they age, their bodies are going to undergo the same changes that all of us experience as we age: metabolism is going to slow, skin is going to lose its elasticity, and fat cells are going to enlarge wherever they are present. If fat cells have been largely removed from everywhere but your butt, then that is where the cumulative effects of the above changes are going to be most seen.

In about 10 years, we are going to see an epidemic of women with dimply butts the size of Volkswagens.

## THOUGHTS ON THE MORTALITY RATE IN THE U.S. FOR BUTT SURGERY?

**Richard Warren:** In 2017, there was an article in *Aesthetic Surgery Journal* entitled "Mortality from Gluteal Fat Grafting: Recommendations from the ASERF Task Force." The report found that, worldwide, the chances of dying from this operation could be as high as 1:2000. That makes it, by a long shot, the most lethal cosmetic operation in plastic surgery.

**Jim Grotting:** With the great surge in interest in buttock enhancement surgery primarily with fat grafting, we have unfortunately seen an uptick in sudden deaths, probably related to fat embolism to the lungs from injury to some of the larger veins around the sciatic nerve. Plastic surgeons are studying this issue intently so as to prevent these complications. No deaths are ever acceptable from an elective cosmetic procedure. Many of these unfortunate deaths have occurred in unregulated clinics by untrained or unscrupulous practitioners. Nevertheless, these unfortunate occurrences reflect poorly on the entire field of aesthetic procedures. We must do everything possible to prevent these tragedies from happening.

## DESCRIBE THE MOST BEAUTIFUL BUTT IN THE WORLD AND WHO'S ELIGIBLE TO GET ONE.

**Armando Soto:** The most beautiful behind in the world looks great in every context and garment, and ages well with the rest of the body. We've all seen the bikini photos of Kim Kardashian, right? I don't think anyone not trying to stay famous for having ridiculous proportions or marry a rapper wants to look like that.

**Ashley Gordon:** There is no one butt that is the most beautiful in the world. Like all things beautiful, it's about balance and proportion.

## MOST EXPENSIVE BUTT PROCEDURES?

**Armando Soto:** In Florida, there are many women who have unfortunately allowed someone to inject them with industrial-grade silicone or other non-medical substances, only to experience severe complications and deformity. These patients require a series of operations to remove the material and then reconstruct the attractive buttocks they desire. This costs between $15,000 and $30,000.

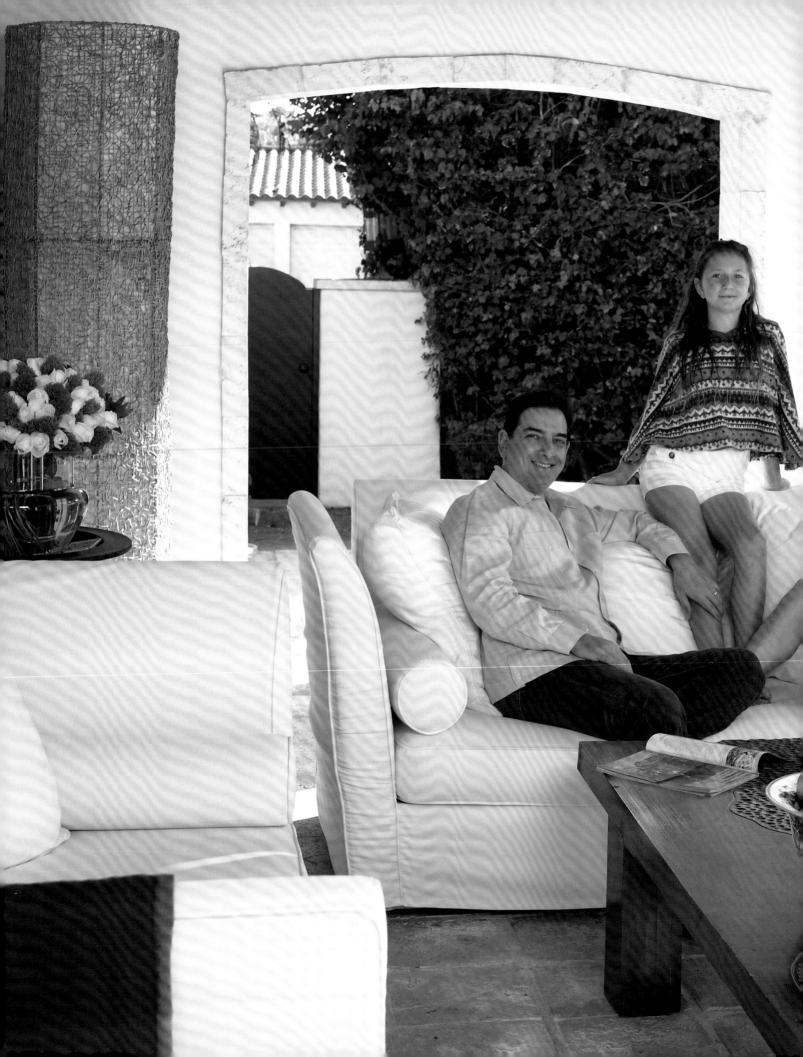

DR. ADAM RUBINSTEIN

# W

HEN PEOPLE MEET A PLASTIC SURGEON IN a social setting, they sometimes feel a bit self-conscious, imagining that the doctor has already sized them up and—at a moment's glance—determined exactly how to "fix" them. Adam Rubinstein's friends appreciate that he only analyzes appearances by request. He admires beauty in all forms, whether it aligns with popular looks or has a uniqueness all its own.

## PLASTIC SURGERY IS NOT ABOUT "NEED"; IT'S ABOUT "WANT."

Yes, Adam is a respected plastic surgeon; yet perhaps even more importantly, he is also a husband, a father of two, and—as one colleague aptly described him—"a true Southern gentleman." Adam's genuine character and sincere regard for the well-being of others are distinguishing elements of his practice.

Adam explains his approach: "There might be something obvious to the world that's not ideal—say a disproportionately large nose or a bulging stomach—but if it doesn't bother that person, then it doesn't deserve discussion." He continues, "I frequently explain to people that plastic surgery is not about 'need'; it's about 'want.' Nobody needs what I do. My patients come to me with their wants, and it's my job to help them make the best choices to achieve their goals safely."

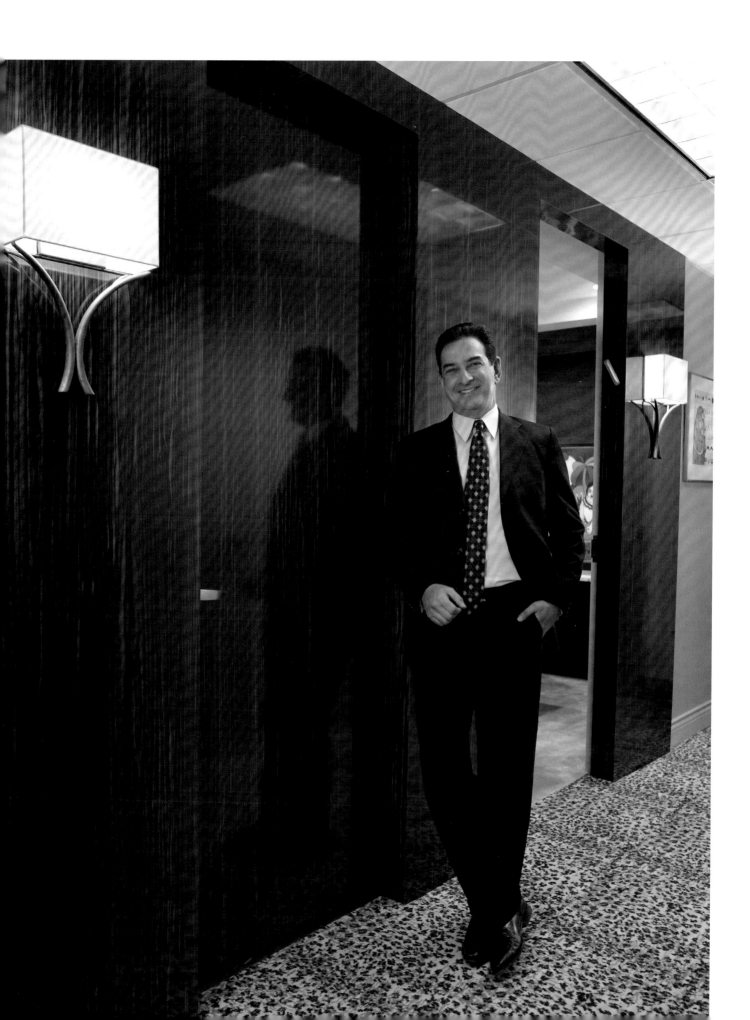

OUT OF RESPECT FOR HIS patients, he never plays the "What would you do for me?" game. Rather, he visits with his patients to figure out what motivates them and what may bring them joy. If he discovers that someone who wants to feel younger actually looks quite young already, he may propose a minimally invasive solution that brilliantly achieves the goal, rather than surgery. And if there isn't enough room for improvement, or a safe and effective way to achieve the patient's goals, he is very comfortable telling that patient "no." He only recommends procedures that will achieve measurable improvements. "Sometimes knowing when to say 'no' is more important than anything else. If I wouldn't recommend something for my wife, brother, or sister, I won't recommend it for my patients." Adam's personal, family-oriented philosophy is certainly unique in the business of beauty.

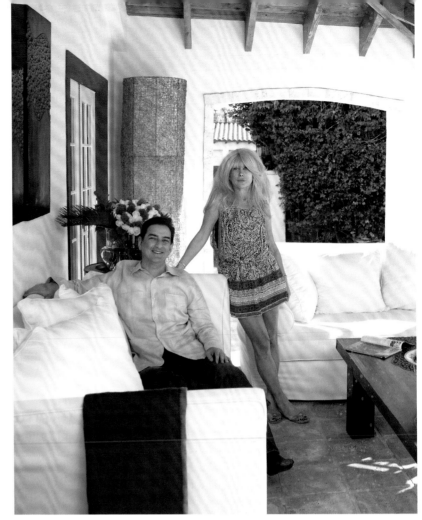

Some doctors like to specialize. Adam prefers a broader approach, because what doesn't work well for one type of procedure might prove groundbreaking in another. Combining best practices, instruments, and perspectives across the spectrum—from breast augmentation to tummy tucks, facelifts, and even nonsurgical procedures—allows him to recommend the absolute best solutions available. It also keeps him at the forefront of the industry, pushing for better, safer, more effective approaches to surgical and cosmetic procedures.

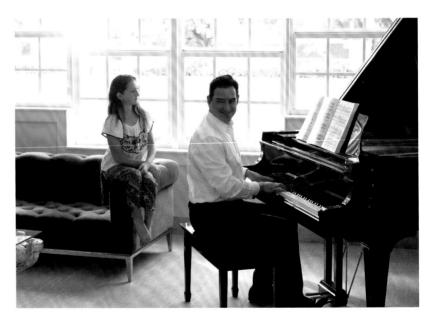

To date, one of Adam's favorite procedures is a brachioplasty (an arm lift)—he calls it an absolute privilege to perform. Technically speaking, his entire profession caters to "wants," not "needs," but this surgery toes the line because it so profoundly changes people's lives. It is the final step of a long journey to achieving significant weight loss of 50 pounds or even hundreds of pounds. As the bandages are removed, patients catch a glimpse of sleek, firm arms—their arms—and the moment is surreal, for this is perhaps the first time in their lives they have experienced the incredibly powerful feeling of being slim. Tears of joy always follow.

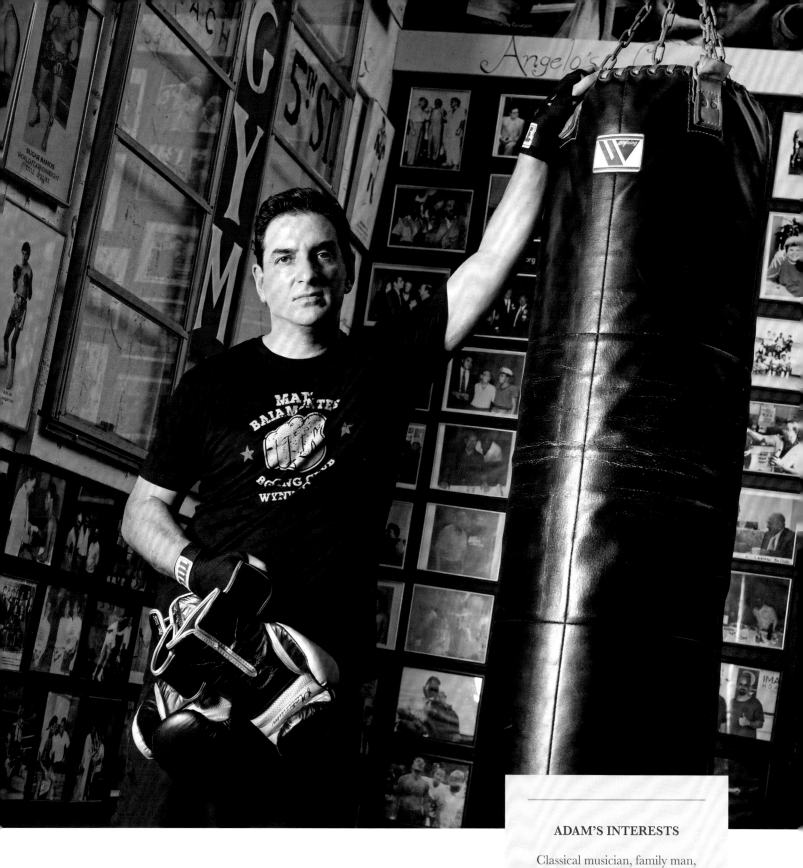

## ADAM'S INTERESTS

Classical musician, family man, and Little League coach, Adam cherishes his annual father-son vacations. Adam and his son plan to visit every baseball stadium in the country, a few memory-making games at a time.

"The truth is we're all fine just the way we are."
Adam Rubinstein

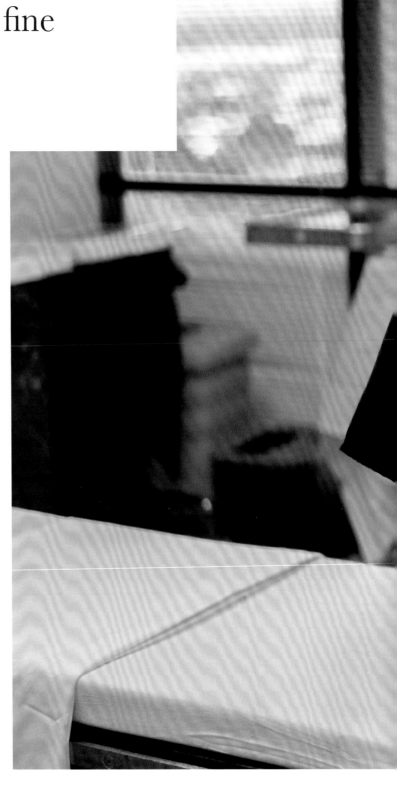

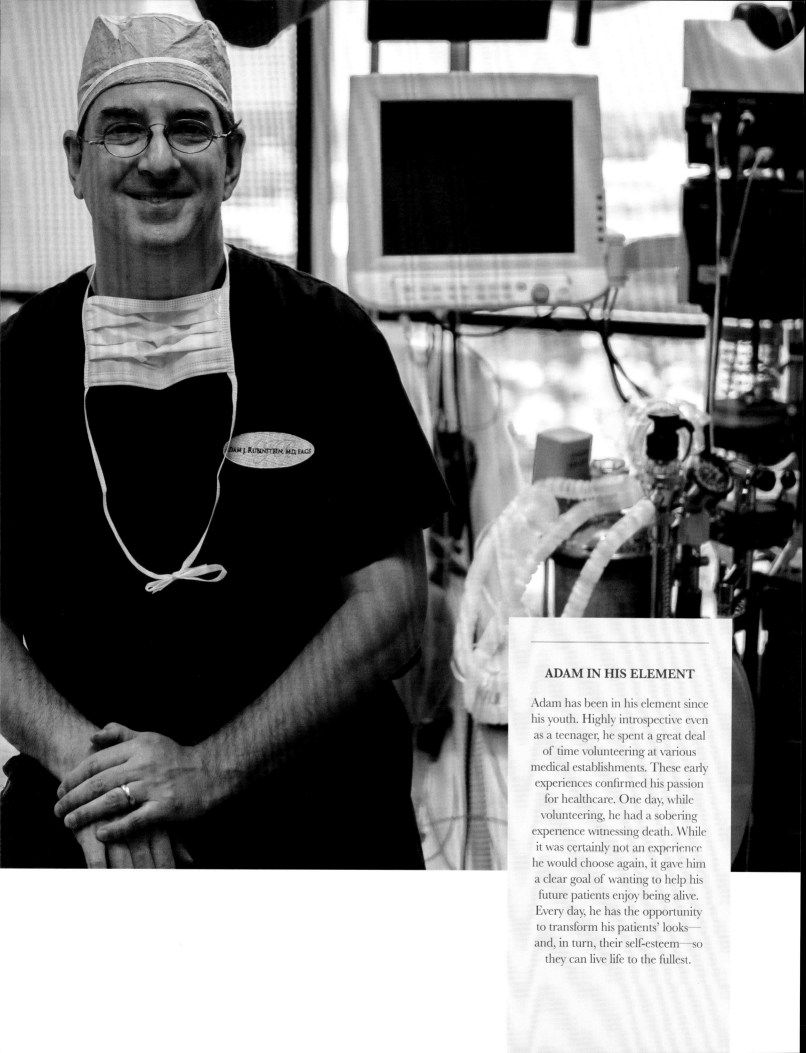

## ADAM IN HIS ELEMENT

Adam has been in his element since his youth. Highly introspective even as a teenager, he spent a great deal of time volunteering at various medical establishments. These early experiences confirmed his passion for healthcare. One day, while volunteering, he had a sobering experience witnessing death. While it was certainly not an experience he would choose again, it gave him a clear goal of wanting to help his future patients enjoy being alive. Every day, he has the opportunity to transform his patients' looks— and, in turn, their self-esteem—so they can live life to the fullest.

"Vaginal rejuvenation has one of the highest rates of patient satisfaction, making women feel more confident and sexy."
Ashley Gordon

REJUVENATION

## WHAT IS THE MOST EFFECTIVE TECHNIQUE FOR VAGINAL REJUVENATION?

**Ashley Gordon:** It's different for every patient, but the most popular surgical procedure is labiaplasty, which contours the labia minora and excess tissue around the clitoris, if present. This procedure has soared in popularity in recent years, and there are a myriad of reasons why women are opting for labiaplasty. The vast majority of my patients have both aesthetic and functional concerns. Sometimes it's something as simple as asymmetry, but usually there is some degree of irritation of the tissues. Excess labial tissues can create rubbing and discomfort, cause issues with hygiene, affect one's sex life, and limit certain types of exercise—not to mention causing discomfort in yoga pants and bathing suits. This procedure has one of the highest rates of patient satisfaction, making women feel more confident and sexy.

**Armando Soto:** This would depend on the patient and her anatomy, but the most effective rejuvenation should pay attention to the vagina itself, as well as the external labia and the patient's symptoms.

**Jennifer Walden:** Currently, treating the vaginal canal with either a radiofrequency device or an ablative laser to rebuild the collagen and mucosal tissue has been the most effective. My practice is conducting a study combining these two modalities to compare the results of using only one device to treat the vaginal canal versus using both to treat both deep and superficial layers.

**Clyde Ishii:** Labiaplasty (reduction of the labia minora) is very effective, as is fat grafting to the labia majora. A plump pubic mons can be contoured with liposuction. The best technique for rejuvenation of the vaginal canal is still under investigation.

## WHAT ARE REALISTIC EXPECTATIONS WITH A VAGINAL REJUVENATION?

**Jennifer Walden:** Patients should expect noticeable improvement. Someone coming in with slight vaginal laxity will usually experience slightly tight to moderately tight results post procedure. We have been pleased with the response in our female clientele.

**Clyde Ishii:** Surgery on the external genitalia (labia minora, majora, mons) can yield very satisfactory results. Surgery to tighten the vagina and rejuvenate the lining is less predictable with today's technology. Some patients may claim significant improvement, while others are less satisfied.

**Armando Soto:** With the most modern treatments involving radiofrequency, I think that well-chosen patients can expect meaningful improvement in symptoms of bladder leakage with sneezing, coughing, or laughing, as well as improvements in external appearance, and improved sexual satisfaction.

**Ashley Gordon:** As with everything, it depends on the individual's situation. Age, genetics, how many children she's had, and the type of delivery can all play a factor. With current technologies, including radiofrequency and lasers, along with precise surgical techniques, we can significantly rejuvenate this area, improving both aesthetics and function.

## DO MULTIPLE VAGINAL REJUVENATION PROCEDURES ENHANCE THE RESULTS, OR IS THERE A LIMIT TO HOW MUCH CAN BE IMPROVED?

**Clyde Ishii:** Labiaplasty and liposuction of a full mons can yield great results with one procedure. On occasion, a minor revision is needed. Plumping up the labia majora with fat may take more than one procedure. Rejuvenation of the vaginal canal usually requires more than one procedure to get the optimal result, but there is a limit to the degree of improvement.

**Armando Soto:** Multiple procedures are usually not necessary to enhance the results, as these are usually excellent with a single treatment. Repeated procedures are recommended in order to maintain the improvement, however.

**Jennifer Walden:** After the first treatment session, which is usually a series of three, patients can maintain results by having a yearly touch-up procedure, which will not necessarily improve upon their initial result, but will increase the longevity. There is a limit due to the natural aging process, child bearing, and hormonal fluctuations, although we are finding that combining an ablative laser with radiofrequency heat indeed enhances outcome.

**Ashley Gordon:** Often a combination approach is best. Labiaplasty is done for external genitalia concerns, and lasers and/or radiofrequency devices are better for internal concerns like laxity, stress-related urinary incontinence, and vaginal dryness.

REJUVENATION

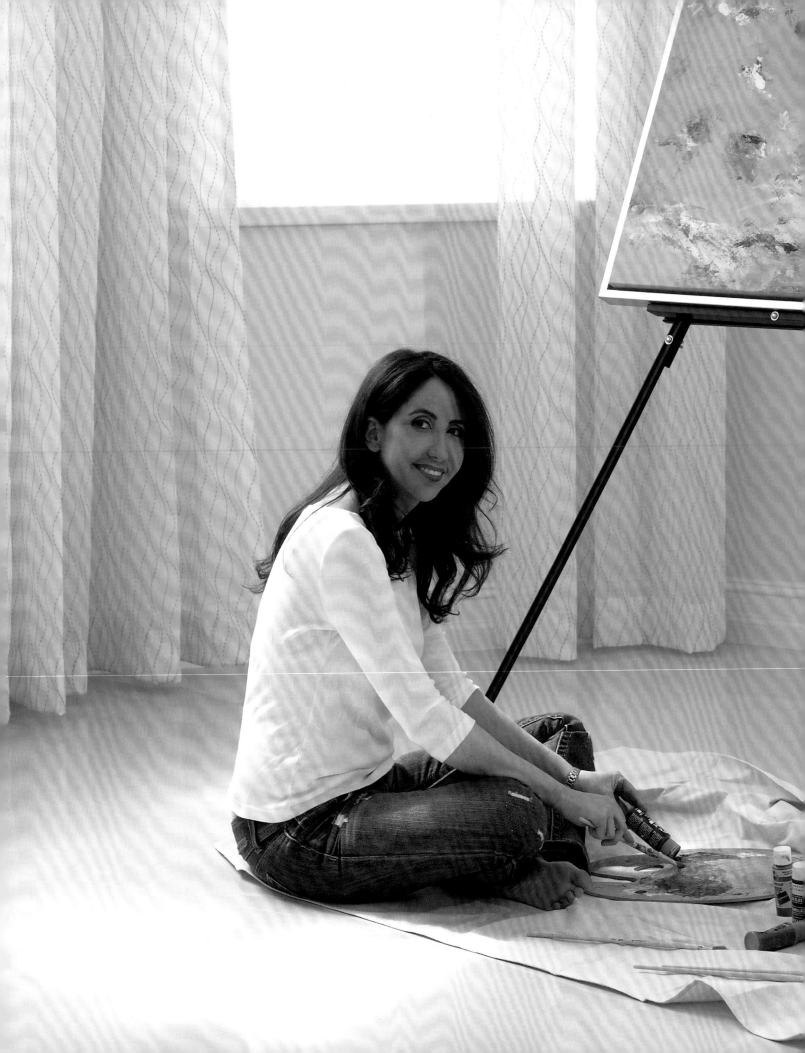

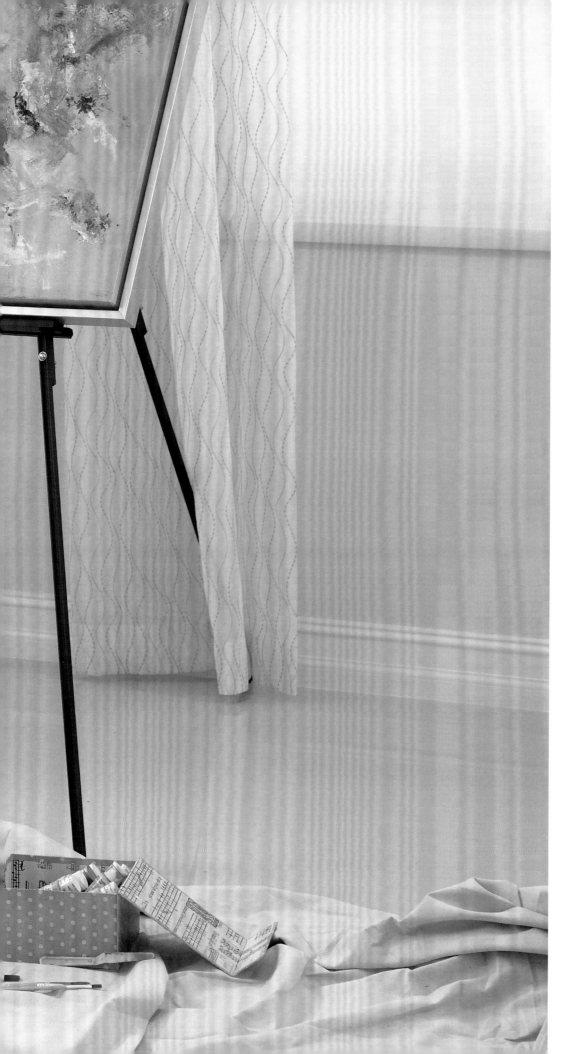

DR. ROBYN SIPERSTEIN-PAUL

R OBYN SIPERSTEIN-PAUL IS FASCINATED WITH THE intrinsic desire to be beautiful. She recognizes that people's motivations to achieve beauty are as varied as how they define beauty. Some want to be perceived as more intelligent to ensure career success. Others seek greater self-confidence. Some just want to change their looks to align with popular culture. And of course there's the eternal quest for the fountain of youth. The desired goal has everything to do with Robyn's approach.

With a lifelong love of learning and orientation toward personal growth, Robyn does a great amount of research in her profession, seeking to push the industry into new realms by finding safer and more effective ways to achieve amazing results. At any given time, she can be found collaborating with an organization or two to conduct trials that breathe excitement into the field of cosmetic dermatology, which is constantly evolving.

Subscribing to a Darwinian perspective, Robyn believes that beauty is both a strategic advantage and an adaptive characteristic. She has long been enamored of the primal notions of beauty—men who are tall, strong, able to provide for their families; women who are youthful, curvaceous, innately maternal.

BEAUTY IS BOTH A STRATEGIC ADVANTAGE AND AN ADAPTIVE CHARACTERISTIC.

While Robyn loves the depth of the topic of beauty, she also appreciates the visual simplicity of beautiful things. Ever inspired by nature, she appreciates the delicate patterns of seashells, the brilliant hues of a sunset on the beach, the clean lines of a perfect circle.

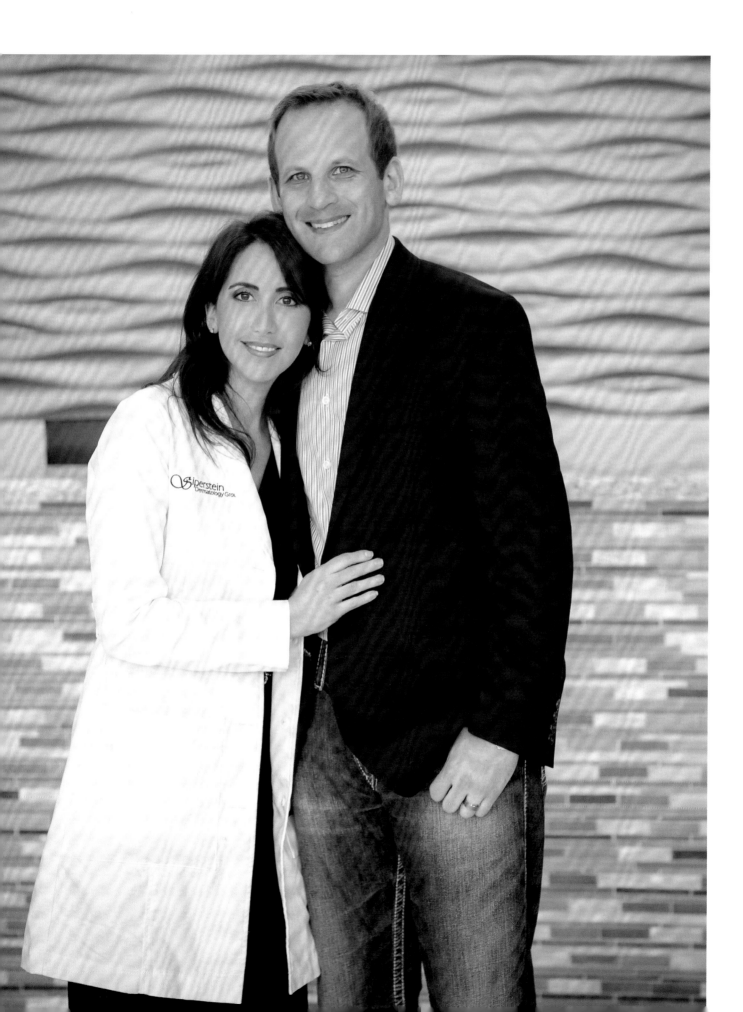

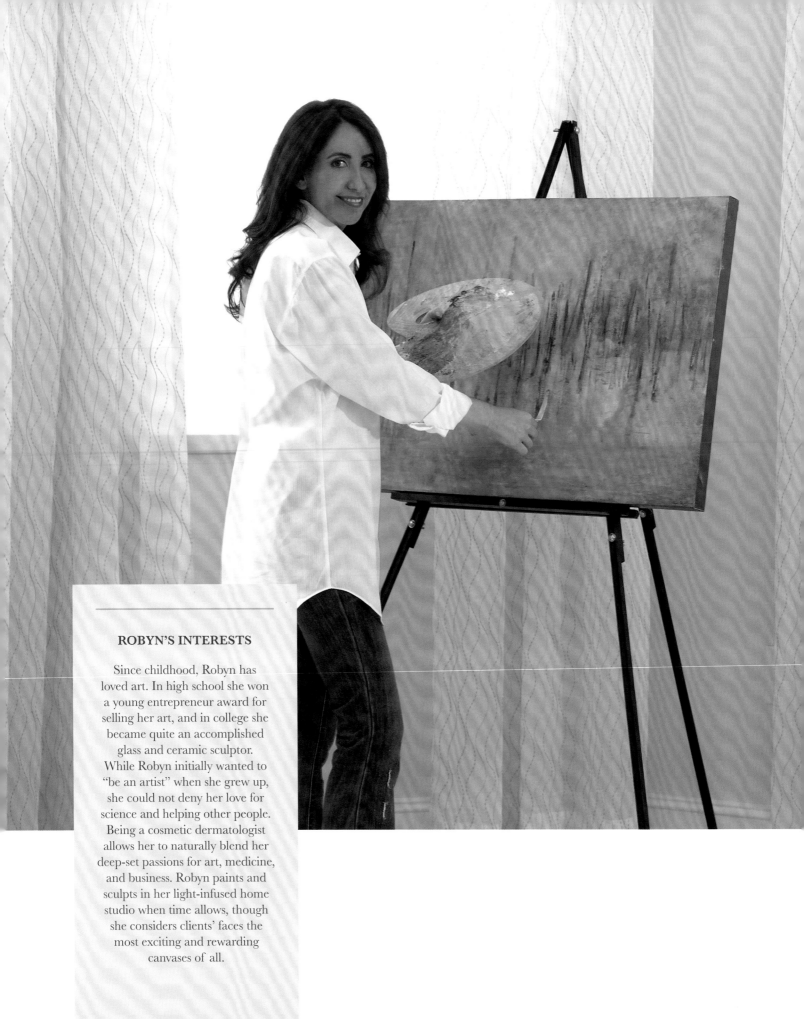

## ROBYN'S INTERESTS

Since childhood, Robyn has loved art. In high school she won a young entrepreneur award for selling her art, and in college she became quite an accomplished glass and ceramic sculptor. While Robyn initially wanted to "be an artist" when she grew up, she could not deny her love for science and helping other people. Being a cosmetic dermatologist allows her to naturally blend her deep-set passions for art, medicine, and business. Robyn paints and sculpts in her light-infused home studio when time allows, though she considers clients' faces the most exciting and rewarding canvases of all.

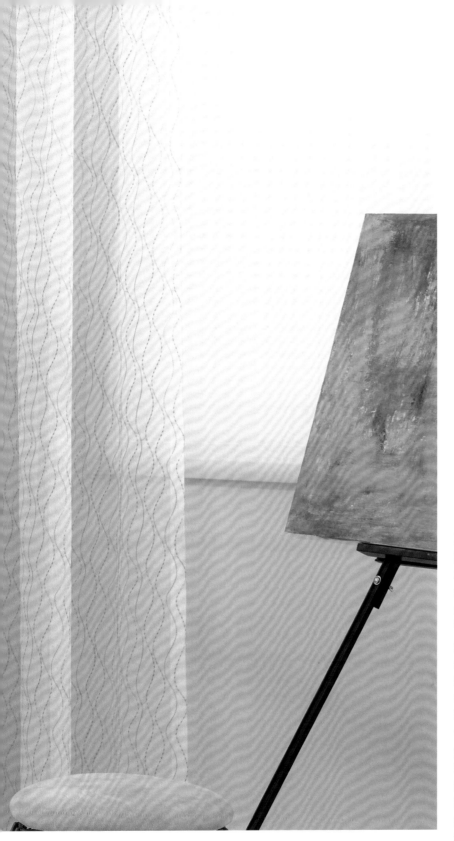

BEAUTY IS SUBJECTIVE, and it's also highly personal and emotional. Robyn is mindful to educate all of her clients on their options—the benefits, the risks, and anything else they should consider. She gives them an "if you were my mom or sister or best friend" professional recommendation and then empowers them to make the decisions that feel right for them. There's one caveat: She knows that she does her best work when she's true to her aesthetic—timeless, elegant, natural. So when a client pulls out a questionable celebrity portrait, Robyn is quick to point out what looks fake in order to deepen the discussion. If the trendy unnatural look is truly desired, Robyn kindly refers a colleague who will be a better match. Her honesty is a breath of fresh air, and it is precisely why clients trust her so completely.

While she entered the profession with a strict medical focus, the inspiring opportunity to enhance not merely skin, but also the way people feel about themselves, was more than enough to lure Robyn into the glamorous world of cosmetic dermatology. She has the pleasure of maximizing her clients' looks so they can achieve their full potential, because right or wrong, being beautiful has its advantages. "I wish everyone in the world could know their own beauty," she graciously declares.

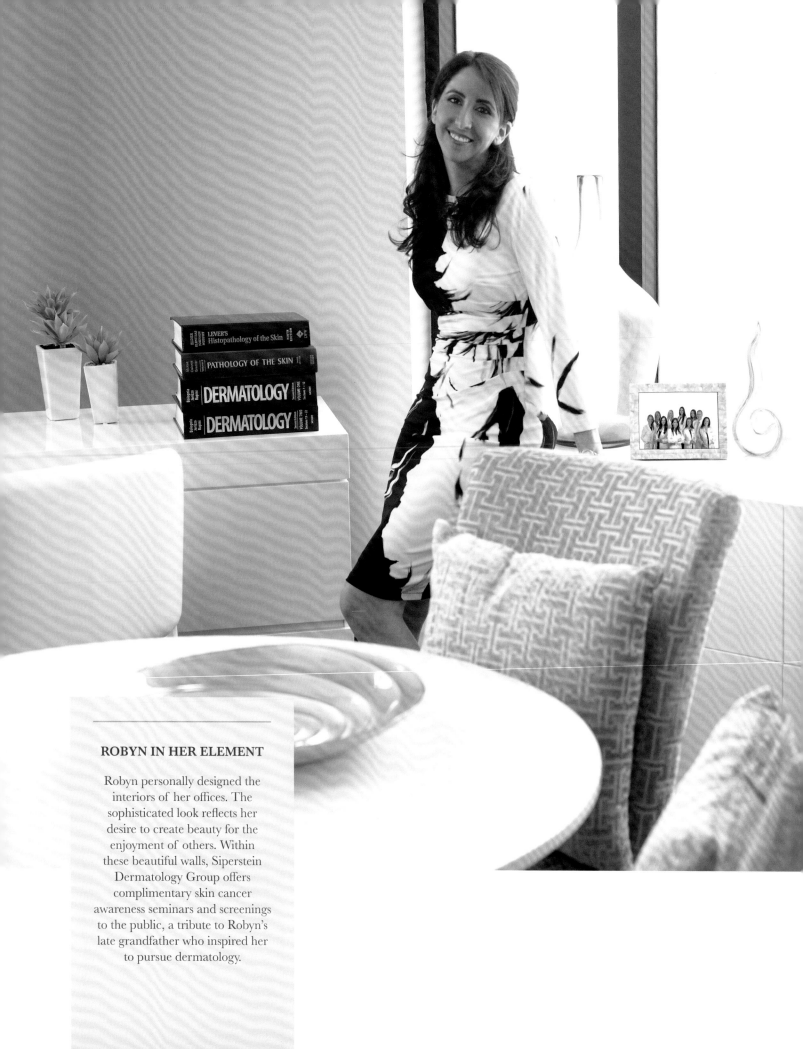

LEVER'S
Histopathology of the Skin

PATHOLOGY OF THE SKIN

DERMATOLOGY

DERMATOLOGY

### ROBYN IN HER ELEMENT

Robyn personally designed the interiors of her offices. The sophisticated look reflects her desire to create beauty for the enjoyment of others. Within these beautiful walls, Siperstein Dermatology Group offers complimentary skin cancer awareness seminars and screenings to the public, a tribute to Robyn's late grandfather who inspired her to pursue dermatology.

"Beauty is anything that gives you pleasure or joy to look at."
Robyn Siperstein-Paul

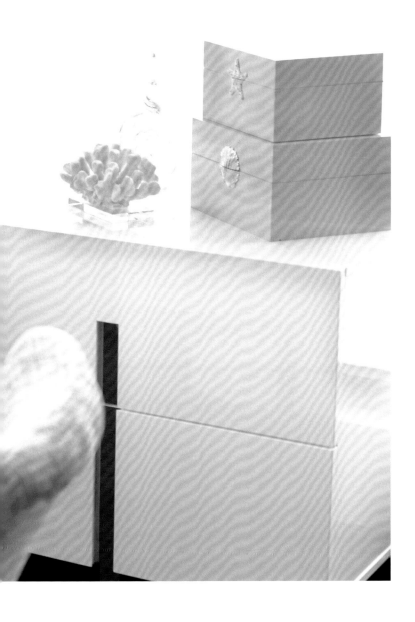

"Being able to say 'no' is the mark of an experienced, ethical surgeon."
Ashley Gordon

# OUTRAGEOUS REQUESTS

**WHEN PATIENTS COME TO YOU WITH UNREASONABLE REQUESTS, WHERE DO YOU DRAW THE LINE, AND HOW DO YOU BREAK THE NEWS THAT THEY WON'T BE BENEFITING FROM YOUR SERVICES?**

**Ashley Gordon:** I draw the line if someone has body dysmorphic disorder, is motivated by the wrong reasons, like trying to save their marriage, or has unrealistic expectations. With the last, I gently explain why their expectations cannot be met because of their current situation (anatomy, tissue quality, genetics, etc.). I explain that their canvas isn't blank, and we have to work with what we have. Most patients understand this once it's explained to them, but some just won't accept that what they want isn't possible. In these cases, I'm very honest and simply tell them that I can't give them the result they are looking for. Being able to say "no" is the mark of an experienced, ethical surgeon.

**Armando Soto:** I always assume two things when visiting with someone for the first time: they want me to keep them safe, and they want to look the best they can. When a patient is asking me for something that I believe is going to compromise either of those priorities, I work very hard to explain to them how their decision making may not be in their best interests. They usually get it, but occasionally I meet someone who is quite determined to proceed down a road I would not recommend for them. At that point I will usually explain that I am concerned for them, because I am sure they will find someone willing to take their money and agree to their choices, but I would not want to be the one they are unhappy with when they realize their error down the road.

**Clyde Ishii:** The doctor-patient relationship is a two-way street, and each party has certain responsibilities. The doctor must be properly trained before treating the patient, inform the patient of available options/associated risks, and treat the patient with respect. Then the patient's request must be reasonable, and his/her expectations must be realistic. If I deem the patient's request to be unreasonable, or if his or her expectations are unrealistic, I gently tell the patient that I do not have the skills to get the result they desire.

**Sheila Nazarian:** I tell them that I don't think I would be able to meet their expectations.

**Charles Thorne:** If the patient's perception of the problem is too far from my perception of it, I suggest to the patient that he or she reconsider. In other words, if the patient talks about his or her nose being hideous or butchered and I think it looks attractive, we are unlikely to be a good match.

**Richard Warren:** In my practice, I find myself saying "no" a lot. A patient's request for cosmetic surgery may be unreasonable for a lot of different reasons: First and foremost, there are many medical problems that will override my willingness to do some cosmetic surgery. Patients are often surprised that we care about such things; but of course, they are looking at real surgery, with real potential problems, so it's a matter of safety first. For example, a patient may have a predisposition to getting DVT (blood clots in the leg) and therefore might not be a candidate for a lengthy abdominoplasty. Often in the facial rejuvenation age group we encounter medical problems like high blood pressure that must be corrected before we can safely proceed with surgery. A difficult type of patient to turn down is the individual who has unrealistic expectations about what surgery can do for them. Technically, they may be a candidate for the surgery, but their concept of what can be accomplished is grossly inflated.

Proceeding to the operating room in that setting is a recipe for disaster, because the surgeon can skillfully do a state-of-the-art operation, but the patient will never be happy with the result. Often the risk/benefit ratio is unreasonable. This situation crops up when the improvement the patient can expect from surgery is minimal, but the surgery they are asking for is complex, with some inherent risks. Yes, it could be done, but ethically, the surgeon may feel that the right thing to do for the patient's wellbeing is not to proceed. Probably the most common reason I say no is the patient just doesn't really need what they are asking for. I do a lot of facial rejuvenation, and often I suggest other alternatives than a facelift, because I think the result from surgery would be too minimal, and therefore that particular patient should wait. In that setting, nonsurgical alternatives will buy the patient time until they are ready for a major operation. How do we turn patients down for surgery? That is actually very easy. Turning a patient down for surgery is simply a matter of telling them the truth. Sometimes they don't like to hear what you have to say, but doing the right thing is always better in the long run.

## MOST OUTRAGEOUS REQUESTS?

**Clyde Ishii:** A 20-year-old male asked me if I could implant a screw in his skull. He wanted to attach a feather to his head and didn't want it to fall off while riding his motorcycle. Needless to say, I declined his request. A 23-year-old male came in with his mother for a cosmetic rhinoplasty consultation. His mother dominated the conversation and asked me if I could make her son look like Keanu Reeves. I kindly declined her request.

**Armando Soto:** I will occasionally be asked to perform a truly extreme breast augmentation or remove ribs to more dramatically enhance a woman's waistline. While these maneuvers are possible, I usually explain to my patient why I would not agree to them: I strongly believe that, both in the short term and in the long term, their plastic surgery experience with me should be something that they look back on as a positive enhancement and without regret. Extreme maneuvers will almost always be regretted by both surgeon and patient at some point.

**Sheila Nazarian:** I had one patient ask me to cut off his earlobes completely. I said no.

**Jim Grotting:** I was asked to make one of my patients look exactly like Elvis Presley to further his career as an impersonator. As flattering as it was for him to believe I could actually do it, I had to decline the request.

**Marta Rendon:** Ultimately the matter isn't that the requests are outrageous; it's usually that they are unrealistic. For instance, when a 65-year-old patient walks into my office with a picture of how they looked 30 years ago or, better yet, a picture of Angelina Jolie's lips, and wants me to replicate that.

**Richard Warren:** Generally, I find my patients to be sensible people who have normal concerns about some physical change they would like to make. However, occasionally I will see a person who has a truly off-the-wall request. A few examples of requests I have had over the years are: to take tissue or body parts from one person and transfer them to another person (I didn't do that); to create breast implants "as big as my head" (I didn't do that either); to use a celebrity's photo as inspiration and make the patient look the same (I never do that); and to remove someone's belly button (for a variety of reasons, I did do that one).

**Tracy Pfeifer:** I really don't get them. I am a normal doctor, and people interested in outrageous results don't bother coming to my office.

**Adam Rubinstein:** I once had a patient call and ask if I could remove all the skin on his fingertips and replace it with skin grafts. I politely answered his questions and gave him an appointment for a consultation. Once we hung up I immediately called the FBI, who, as you might imagine, were very interested in meeting this patient. They staked out the office on the day of the consultation, but the patient never showed.

OUTRAGEOUS REQUESTS

"Turning a patient down for surgery is simply a matter of telling them the truth."

Richard Warren

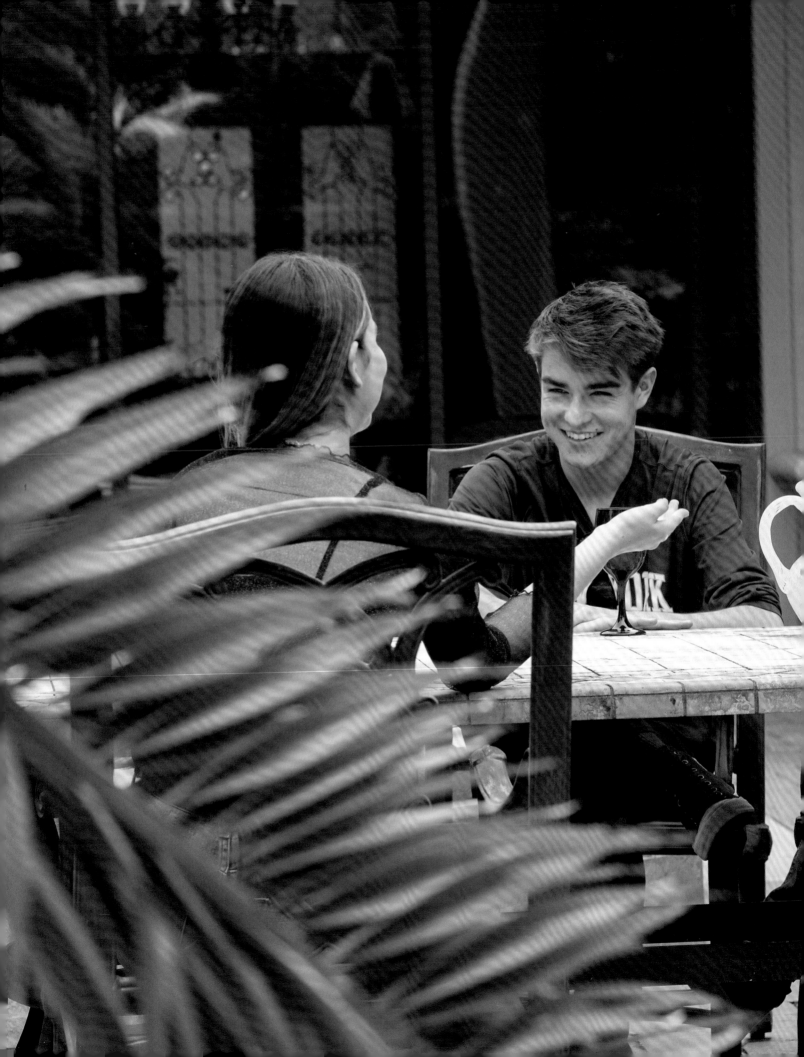

DR. ARMANDO SOTO

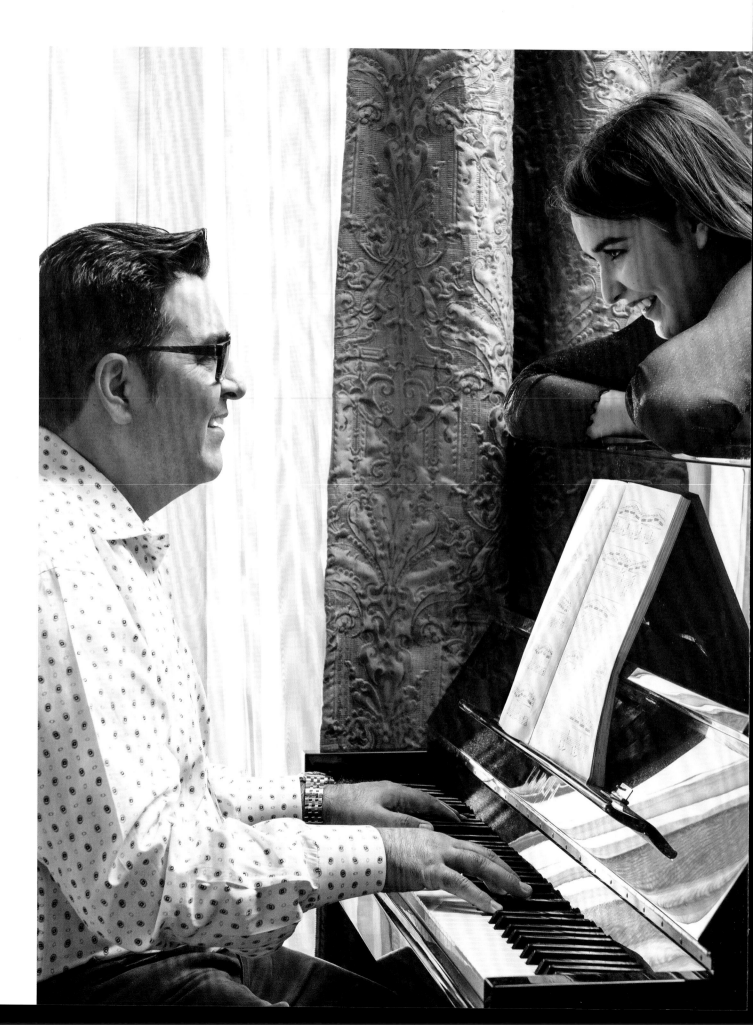

W HEN IT COMES TO WOMEN, Armando Soto has unique depth in his compassion and understanding. He has a wife and a daughter, and he grew up surrounded by women: his mother, four sisters, and aunts galore. Perhaps even more relevant than his comfort in the company of women is the sincere joy he finds in listening to, visiting, and developing professional relationships with his patients in order to make their lives even better.

Armando appreciates that all of his patients—women and men—have different goals, and discovering how to best achieve those goals gives him great pleasure. He respects what they wish to change as well as that with which they are content. He explains, "If a woman says she wants to age gracefully and never do anything to her face, I am thrilled for her, and I say congratulations on achieving that sense of self."

Over the years, Armando has been inspired by seeing patients who wear their imperfections well and simply desire a noninvasive freshening of their looks. He has seen plenty more who find joy beyond measure when he is able to surgically change their looks to match their personal ideals of beauty. When he sees that something is keeping a patient from being happy, he feels compelled to do everything in his power to right the situation—it's an almost-primal response.

> IT'S INSPIRING TO SEE PATIENTS WHO WEAR THEIR IMPERFECTIONS WELL AND SIMPLY DESIRE A NONINVASIVE FRESHENING OF THEIR LOOKS.

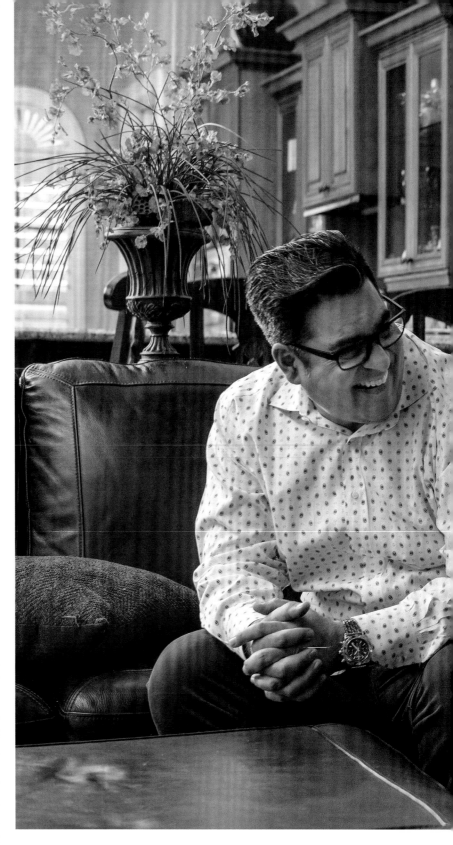

TO ARMANDO, aesthetic medicine is about helping people find peace and balance along the spectrum of internal and external beauty. Those with internal beauty are generally well adjusted individuals who have a calm respect for their fellow travelers in life. Those with outward beauty possess an appearance that is aesthetically, symmetrically, and proportionally pleasing. From Armando's seasoned perspective, the highest form of beauty is "total beauty," which he describes as having achieved harmony between perception of self and actual appearance.

The psychology of beauty is of great interest to Armando because he believes in working toward whatever ideal his patients consider beautiful—within reason, of course. This is a more complex approach than simply applying a singular standard to all of his patients; yet by his measure, it is the right thing to do.

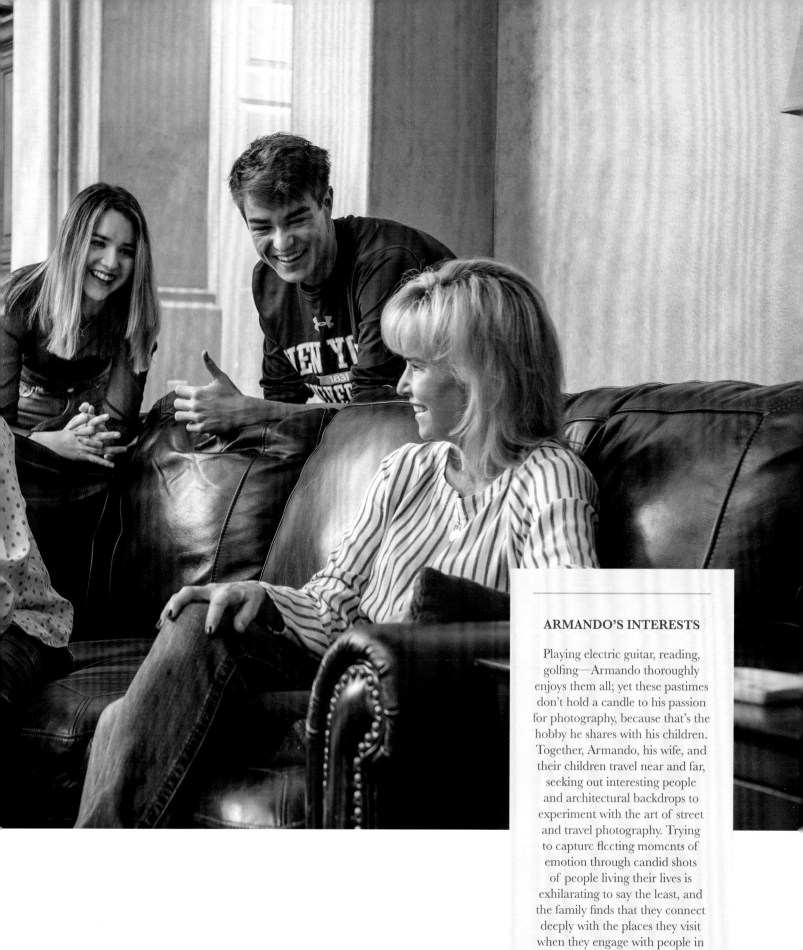

## ARMANDO'S INTERESTS

Playing electric guitar, reading, golfing—Armando thoroughly enjoys them all; yet these pastimes don't hold a candle to his passion for photography, because that's the hobby he shares with his children. Together, Armando, his wife, and their children travel near and far, seeking out interesting people and architectural backdrops to experiment with the art of street and travel photography. Trying to capture fleeting moments of emotion through candid shots of people living their lives is exhilarating to say the least, and the family finds that they connect deeply with the places they visit when they engage with people in such a real way.

"Aesthetic medicine is about helping patients see themselves the way they imagine themselves to be."
Armando Soto

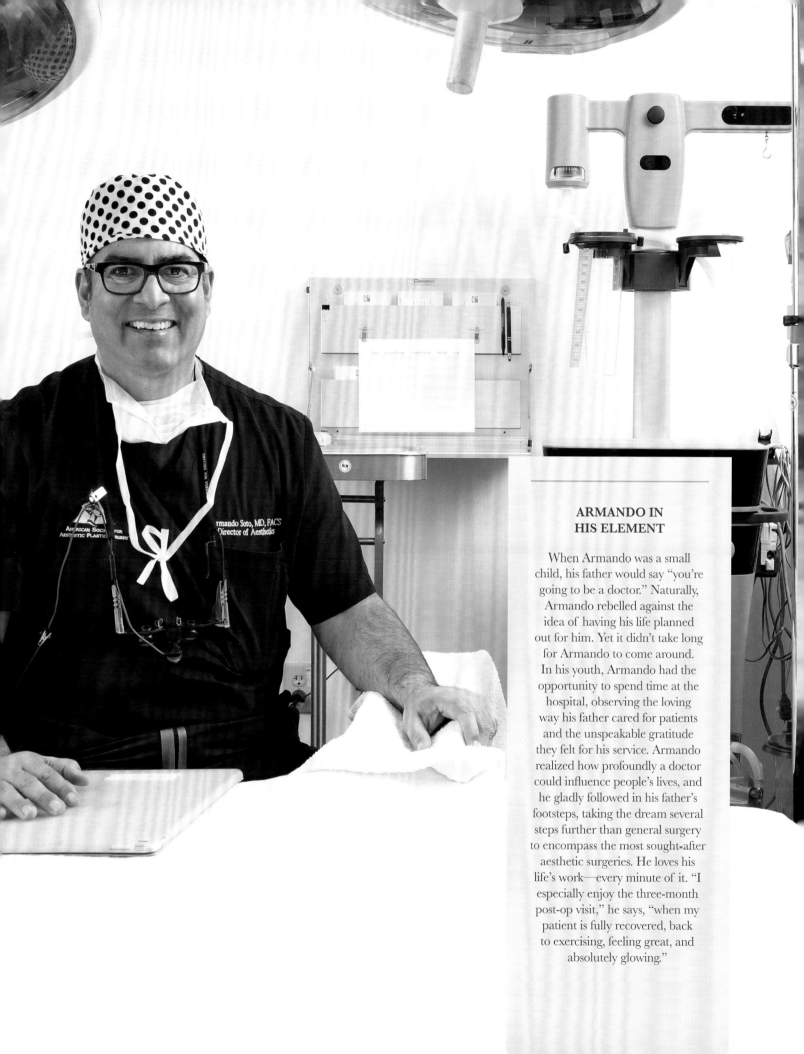

## ARMANDO IN HIS ELEMENT

When Armando was a small child, his father would say "you're going to be a doctor." Naturally, Armando rebelled against the idea of having his life planned out for him. Yet it didn't take long for Armando to come around. In his youth, Armando had the opportunity to spend time at the hospital, observing the loving way his father cared for patients and the unspeakable gratitude they felt for his service. Armando realized how profoundly a doctor could influence people's lives, and he gladly followed in his father's footsteps, taking the dream several steps further than general surgery to encompass the most sought-after aesthetic surgeries. He loves his life's work—every minute of it. "I especially enjoy the three-month post-op visit," he says, "when my patient is fully recovered, back to exercising, feeling great, and absolutely glowing."

"Seeing an introverted, self-conscious individual emotionally blossom after cosmetic surgery feels like a monumental achievement."
Richard Warren

MEMORABLE PATIENTS

## MOST REWARDING EXPERIENCE IN YOUR CAREER?

**Armando Soto:** I find great joy and fulfillment in the patients for whom we are able to provide a true transformation in the way they present themselves to the world. Notable examples would include an 18-year-old woman who did not develop a breast on one side and was severely stunted socially as a result. When I met her, she wouldn't even make eye contact, despite the fact that she was a beautiful girl with a great future. Her parents were equally distressed over the pain their daughter was experiencing. We undertook a two-stage reconstruction resulting in almost perfect symmetry with the other side over about 10 months. She went on to college the confident, easy-smiling, engaging, and beautiful young woman she saw herself to be. Another patient is one who lost 120 pounds over five years through hard work and discipline. When we met, she was swimming in skin, and her marriage was suffering. She had conquered the obesity but felt defeated by the resulting skin. After the body lift, she sent me a photo collage of herself wearing tight jeans and bikini bathing suits, and smiling on adventures with her husband, enjoying a life she never would have even pursued.

**Marta Rendon:** A patient with significant scarring after brain surgery had significant asymmetry of her face. She was extremely depressed and had not gone out of her house in years. After four procedures—a combination of fillers, toxins, and lasers—we were able to give balance to her face, and she started crying when she looked at herself in the mirror.

**Robyn Siperstein-Paul:** A patient had radiation treatments for breast cancer that left her with unsightly blood vessels on her chest. Once I removed them with a laser treatment, she came back with a v-neck shirt—something she hadn't been able to do for five years—crying tears of joy; she finally felt cancer-free, because I'd removed the last reminders of her previous illness.

**Adam Rubinstein:** Early in my career I had a patient who was a young girl; she and two other girls had been playing chicken on a jet ski with three young boys on another jet ski. Unfortunately, neither the boys nor girls flinched. My patient was ejected and flew face-first into the large wooden post on a dock. She had horrible injuries, including the loss of one eye. I collaborated with ophthalmology and neurosurgery in multiple procedures, one lasting about 16 hours, to reconstruct her face. She did very well and is a beautiful young woman today. She sent a lovely thank you card years later that I keep to this day. I still carry her photo in my instrument case as a reminder.

**Richard Warren:** In cosmetic surgery, the most rewarding experience is to witness a personality that is changed for the better, all because of an operation we did. Seeing an introverted, self-conscious individual emotionally blossom after cosmetic surgery feels like a monumental achievement. I can think of several people whom I have seen transformed in this way. One young lady I remember well had a large hooked-shaped nose that made her very self-conscious. She had trouble looking me in the eye. However, behind that nose I could see a beautiful girl with some specific nasal features that are impossible to create surgically, like perfectly shaped small nostrils and porcelain skin. The rhinoplasty I did for her was transformative. In the months afterward, she arrived at my office dressing differently, walking differently, and looking right at me when she spoke. A few years later that same girl entered a very prestigious beauty contest, and she won! From there she went on to a successful professional career that I attribute, at least in part, to the increased confidence my nose operation gave her. It changed her life.

**Ashley Gordon:** Breast reduction in a 14-year-old who was withdrawn, depressed, and anxious about the size of her very large breasts that had been growing since she was 10. She didn't want to go to school or participate in sports or extracurricular activities, and she dreaded the summer. At her initial consultation, she would only let me examine one breast at a time because she was so embarrassed and shy. I had several consultations with her and her parents, as 14 is very young for a breast reduction; but I could see the significant negative impact it was having on her self-esteem and sense of self. We decided together that although she was likely to continue growing and would possibly need a further reduction in the future, doing surgery sooner rather than later was the right choice because of the positive impact it would have on her during this critical time of development. The surgery completely transformed her—physically, emotionally, and mentally—into an active, outgoing, and confident young lady. I was impressed with her parents for their sensitivity in recognizing what she was going through and not just dismissing her concerns and withdrawn behavior as "a teenage phase."

**Tracy Pfeifer:** A patient had multiple breast surgeries involving augmentation and mastopexy. She healed poorly and had a terrible result after multiple, expensive surgeries. She spent a fortune. She was and is a very nice, down-to-earth person. She was told multiple times it was her fault that she did not heal properly. I performed revision-augmentation, and her breasts looked normal again. Not perfect, but much, much better. She was so appreciative, and it really changed her life. She regained her confidence, and everyone noticed this. She started dating again. I see her every year; it's been 10 years now, and she always takes care to remind me how much she appreciates everything we did for her. In a situation like this, it is not just about creating breasts that look pretty; it is the transformation of the entire person on a very fundamental level, a renewing of their spirit and energy. This is the power of cosmetic surgery.

**Clyde Ishii:** I did multiple reconstructive procedures on a young girl who nearly lost her leg when she fell victim to flesh-eating bacteria at age five. She remained upbeat and very positive throughout her multiple operations. She refused to let the tragedy get her down and would wiggle when I examined her, so I called her my Wiggle Worm. She went on to become a beauty queen in Hawaii, and I am certain she will do great things in life.

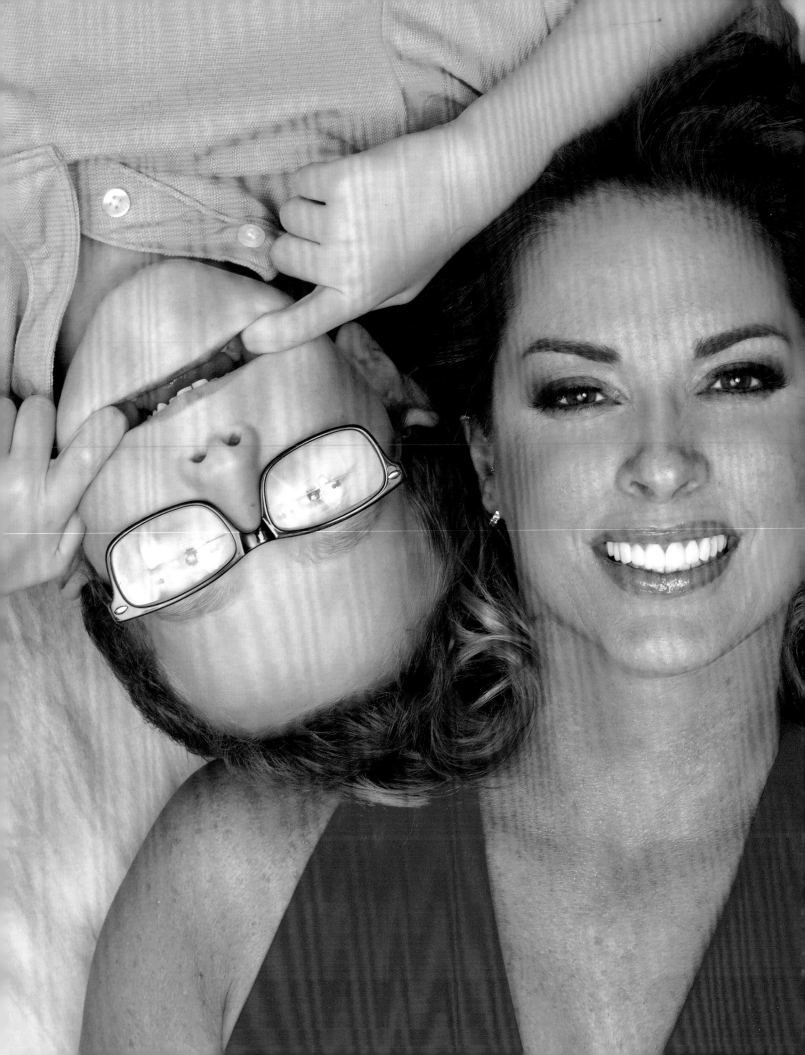

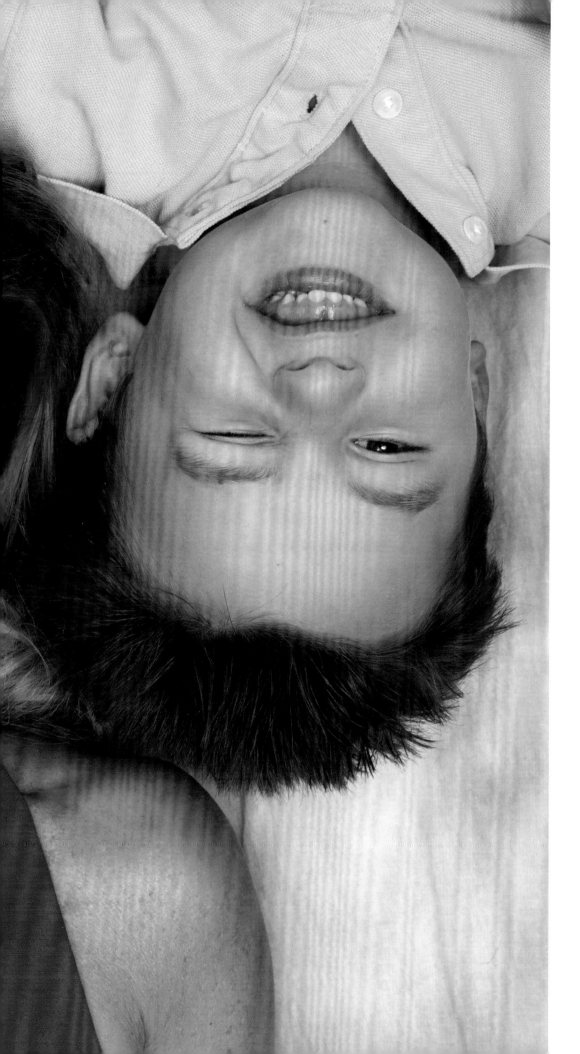

DR. JENNIFER WALDEN

O FTENTIMES A WOMAN'S TOUCH is required for prospective patients to feel comfortable talking about personal topics like vaginal rejuvenation, labiaplasty, and breast augmentation. Jennifer Walden is inspired by the incredibly broad demographic attracted to such procedures—from 20-somethings looking to spice things up, to new moms wanting their bodies back, to grandmothers in their 70s desiring a fresh image. Sure, some patients are vain, and rightly so; but most are not; they are ordinary people with real needs and wants.

## MOST PATIENTS ARE ORDINARY PEOPLE WITH REAL NEEDS AND WANTS.

As a plastic surgeon, Jennifer appreciates the life-changing results that her surgeries create. As a mother, she knows exactly what it's like to love your little ones to the moon and back, and yet wish like anything that you could turn back time for your body's sake. She has great empathy for every mother who wants her tummy, nose, skin, and other uniquely affected areas to be as they once were. Through a combination of surgical and noninvasive procedures, she has helped countless women restore their bodies, confidence, and joy in life.

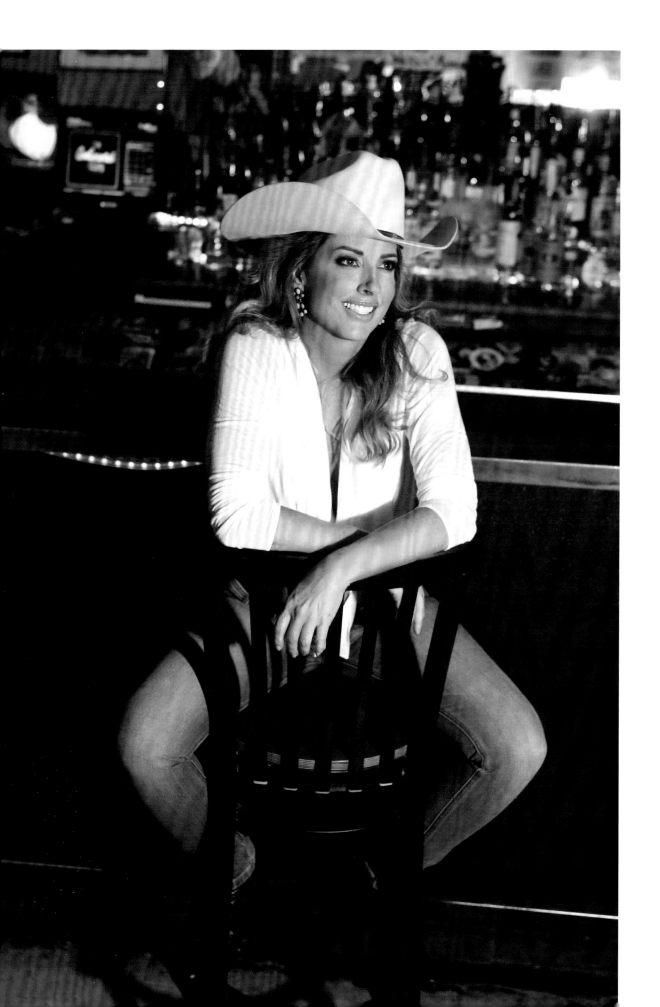

JENNIFER IS INVIGORATED by the highly subjective concept of beauty and loves the process of individualizing her patients' ideas. Her personal aesthetic is natural—not too harsh; nice and timeless—yet she is certainly familiar with the many lenses that form a patient's inclinations. Age, ethnicity, gender, current trends—all of these facets and more influence how people think of themselves and the image they wish to present to the world. She works with men and women of all ages to develop a plan that maximizes their natural beauty.

Continual advancements in the field of cosmetic surgery mean that procedures are more accessible than ever. Jennifer is leading the way as the inventor of several surgical tools, a consultant to top aesthetic companies, a Fellow of the American College of Surgeons, and board member and communications commissioner for the American Society for Aesthetic Plastic Surgery. And in her spare time, she regularly lends her expertise and voice to various public news sources and scholarly journals. She proudly partners with others at the top of the profession to steer the industry in healthy directions.

Just a decade ago, before Jennifer relocated her practice from New York City to Austin, fat transfers were rather uncommon; now the technique is regarded as a safe and effective option for enhancing breasts, facial features, and more. Liposuction is still a mainstay; yet fat melting and fat reduction are also great options. Radiofrequency skin tightening, lasers that destroy fat cells in minutes through a simple-to-use medical belt, vaginal rejuvenation with devices that are nonsurgical, quick, and painless—these breakthroughs are tremendously exciting to this plastic surgeon growing a medspa for noninvasive and minimally invasive procedures. She is always abreast of the latest techniques and at the forefront of exploring the possibilities.

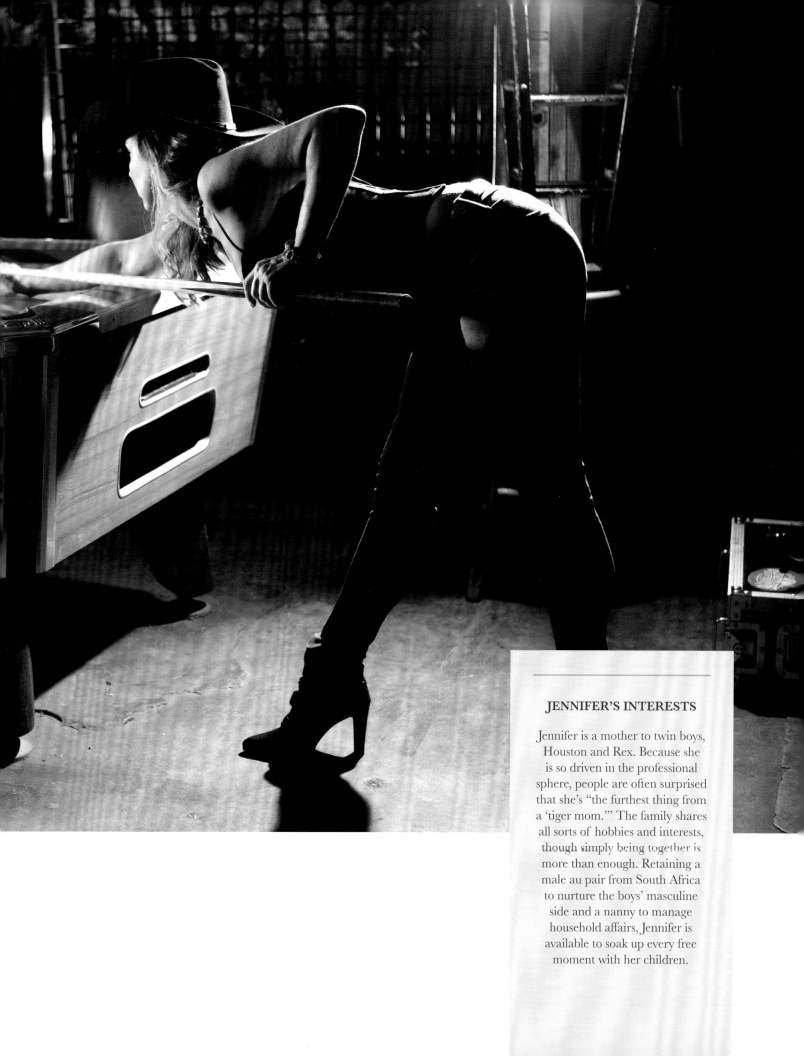

### JENNIFER'S INTERESTS

Jennifer is a mother to twin boys, Houston and Rex. Because she is so driven in the professional sphere, people are often surprised that she's "the furthest thing from a 'tiger mom.'" The family shares all sorts of hobbies and interests, though simply being together is more than enough. Retaining a male au pair from South Africa to nurture the boys' masculine side and a nanny to manage household affairs, Jennifer is available to soak up every free moment with her children.

"Appearance is real. It affects us all, especially as we notice ourselves aging. What a privilege it is to be able to restore appearances so people can feel right again—or right for the first time in their lives."
Jennifer Walden

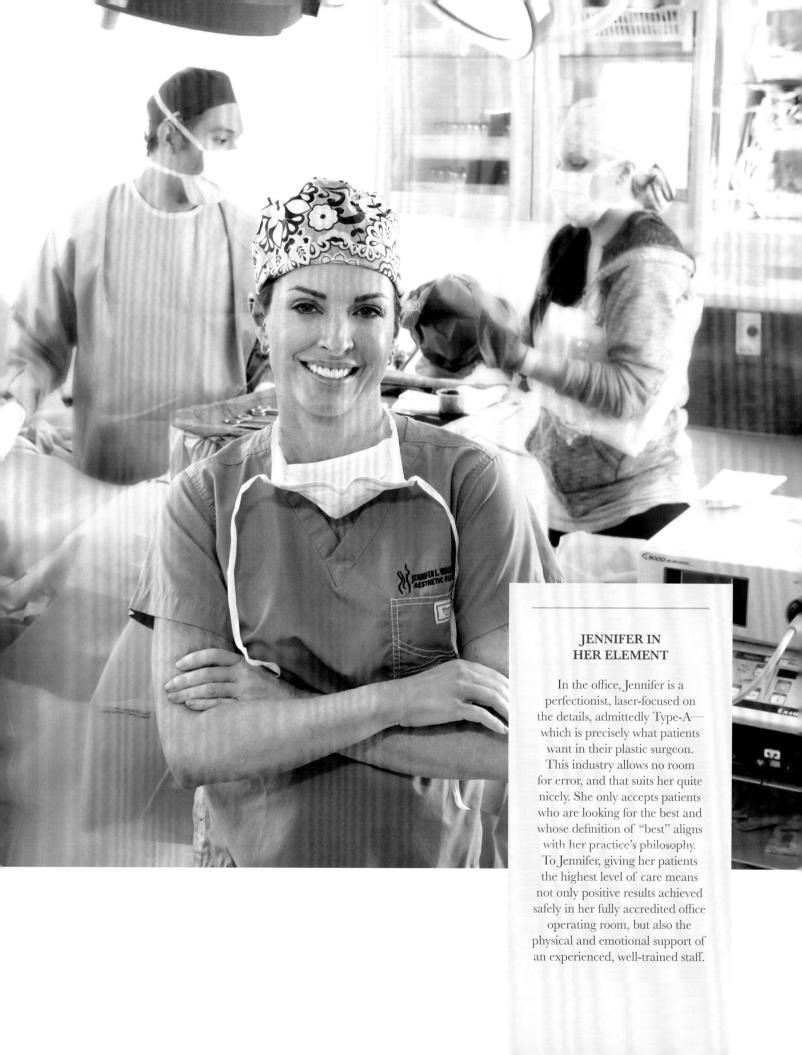

### JENNIFER IN HER ELEMENT

In the office, Jennifer is a perfectionist, laser-focused on the details, admittedly Type-A—which is precisely what patients want in their plastic surgeon. This industry allows no room for error, and that suits her quite nicely. She only accepts patients who are looking for the best and whose definition of "best" aligns with her practice's philosophy. To Jennifer, giving her patients the highest level of care means not only positive results achieved safely in her fully accredited office operating room, but also the physical and emotional support of an experienced, well-trained staff.

"There have been so many advancements in noninvasive procedures in the last five years, I can't wait to see what the future holds!"
Sheila Nazarian

# LOOKING AHEAD

## WHAT DOES THE INDUSTRY LOOK LIKE IN 10 YEARS?

**Richard Warren:** In 10 years, I think we will have seen a steady increase in the public's acceptance of cosmetic procedures and along with that, a steady growth in this field. There will be a greater number and more variety of surgical and nonsurgical procedures being offered. In the surgical arena, we will probably see improvements in fat graft survival, improvements in the control of breast implant capsular contracture, and a steady improvement in surgical methods to rejuvenate the aging face. In the nonsurgical arena, we will likely see improvement in skin tightening technologies, stem cell stimulation, and volume fillers. One concerning issue is the selfie culture. The coming generations have grown up with multiple images of themselves and with exposure to all our new cosmetic interventions. This could lead to many more patients seeking cosmetic surgery that is frivolous and unnecessary.

**Anna Petropoulos:** I believe that the view that I espoused and brought into the industry 20 years ago is becoming more and more mainstream every year that goes by: namely, that technology is increasingly able to prevent surgery or replace it. Isn't it strange that I was ridiculed back then by my surgeon peers, who said these were "foufou" treatments, and that only surgery was worthwhile. Now today, even the most hard-core surgeons are trying to acquire knowledge about noninvasive treatments and begin to utilize them due to their effectiveness and also due to public demand in avoiding surgery.

**Armando Soto:** We are going to be even more strongly focused on maintaining youthful appearance and function, and even less on restoration of the same. I think we will continue to get better at devising and performing noninvasive and minimally invasive treatments that we initiate at younger ages (20 to 30) to prevent the signs of aging.

**Adam Rubinstein:** There have been a lot of advancements in minimally invasive and noninvasive techniques and technology over the last few years. That trend will continue with new technology providing options to achieve great results without surgery.

**Clyde Ishii:** More physicians of all specialties doing cosmetic surgery because it is an unregulated industry. The government is unlikely to step in and regulate it because it wants to avoid restriction of trade at all cost. Noninvasive treatments will be much more advanced. Skin tightening by lasers and other 510(k) devices will be much more effective. Noninvasive modalities will remain very popular but will never totally replace surgery.

**Charles Thorne:** Hopefully the myth that fillers can lift the face will disappear.

**Tracy Pfeifer:** I hope that more patients will realize that cosmetic surgery is important and not to be taken lightly. I hope that we will be able to eliminate people posing as doctors and reduce the number of unqualified persons performing cosmetic surgery. Unfortunately, I think we are heading in the opposite direction.

**Ashley Gordon:** I'm most excited about regenerative medicine using stem cells, because the possibilities are endless, and we are just on the cusp of understanding the various conditions we can treat with these cells. With regenerative medicine, we can harness the body's own powers to heal itself rather than relying on drugs, surgery, or fillers. Most regenerative medicine includes therapies that isolate stem cells and use other cellular products such as PRP (platelet-rich plasma) and growth factors. While there are various sources of stem cells in our bodies, the most abundant numbers are found in our fat. For all of these years, we've been throwing fat away after liposuction, not knowing the regenerative powers of the cells held within it. Stem cells are very complex; but simply put, they serve as a sort of internal repair system. They regularly divide to repair and replace worn out or diseased tissue. They differ from all other cells in the body because they have unique properties: they are capable of dividing and renewing themselves for long periods of time, and they are unspecialized but have the ability to give rise to specialized cell types if needed, like muscle cells or nerve cells. With increasing understanding, we now have technology that makes it easy to extract and isolate the stem cells, all in a single setting. We are currently using it in patients with hair loss to reactivate hair follicles that have gone dormant and also for a variety of skin conditions like hyperpigmentation, wrinkles, scars, burns, and volume loss. The applications are endless, and multiple clinical trials are happening across the country to treat a variety of conditions like congestive heart failure, Parkinson's disease, auto-immune diseases, and joint problems.

"We are going to be even more strongly focused on maintaining youthful appearance and function, and even less on restoration of the same."
Armando Soto

LOOKING AHEAD

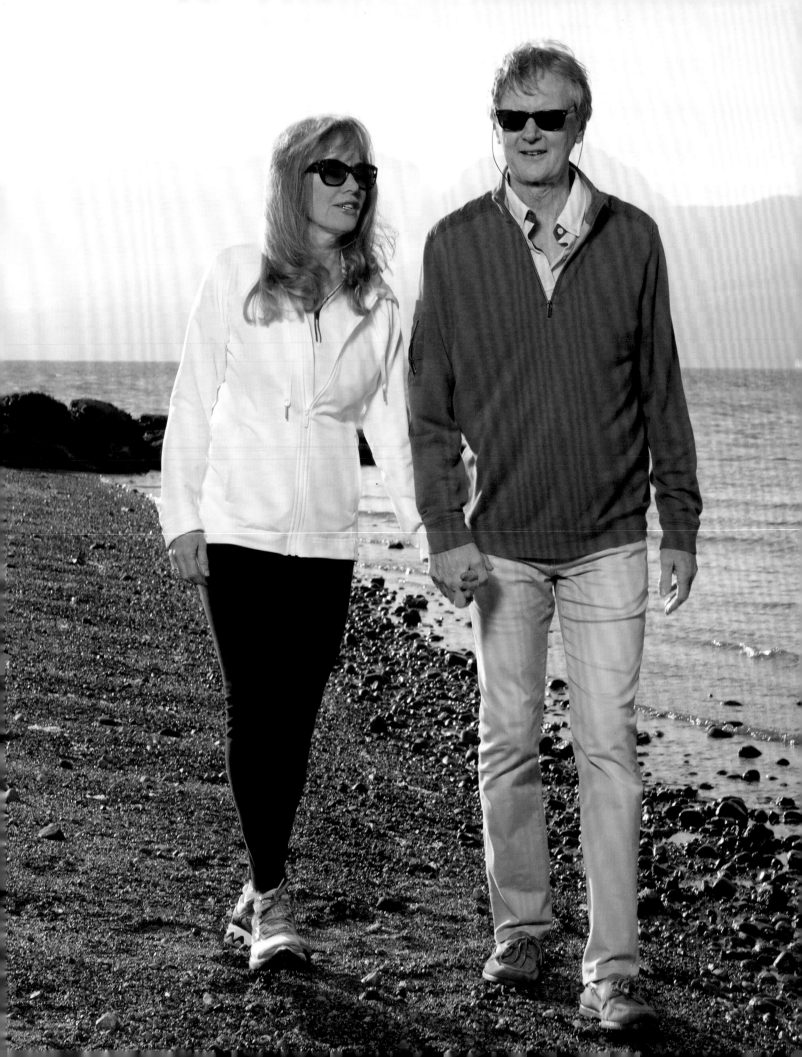

DR. RICHARD J. WARREN

W HEN RICHARD WARREN'S CHILDREN lived at home, he cleared his office calendar for an entire month, every summer, so they could spend meaningful time together at their lake house. He and his wife, Betty, have their priorities straight. When patients come to see Richard, he enjoys the process of helping them figure out their priorities, explaining how realistic their requests are—or aren't—and developing surgical plans to safely achieve their goals.

Over the years, Richard's patients have aged right along with him, "for better or worse," he quips. Many patients who had body surgery decades ago are now electing for facial rejuvenation, and there's no better compliment for a surgeon. Whatever the reason for their visit, patients are met with the same types of questions, geared to draw out their innermost motivations. Richard needs to know precisely why they seek his expertise so that he can determine the best course of treatment. He elaborates, "Cosmetic surgery is invasive, it's serious business. We take a patient's face or body apart and have to put it back together even better than it was. We're working with the art and science of cosmetic surgery but also dealing with the science of patients' minds, so it's imperative to really understand who they are and what they want out of life."

> WE'RE DEALING WITH THE SCIENCE OF PATIENTS' MINDS, SO IT'S IMPERATIVE TO REALLY UNDERSTAND WHO THEY ARE AND WHAT THEY WANT OUT OF LIFE.

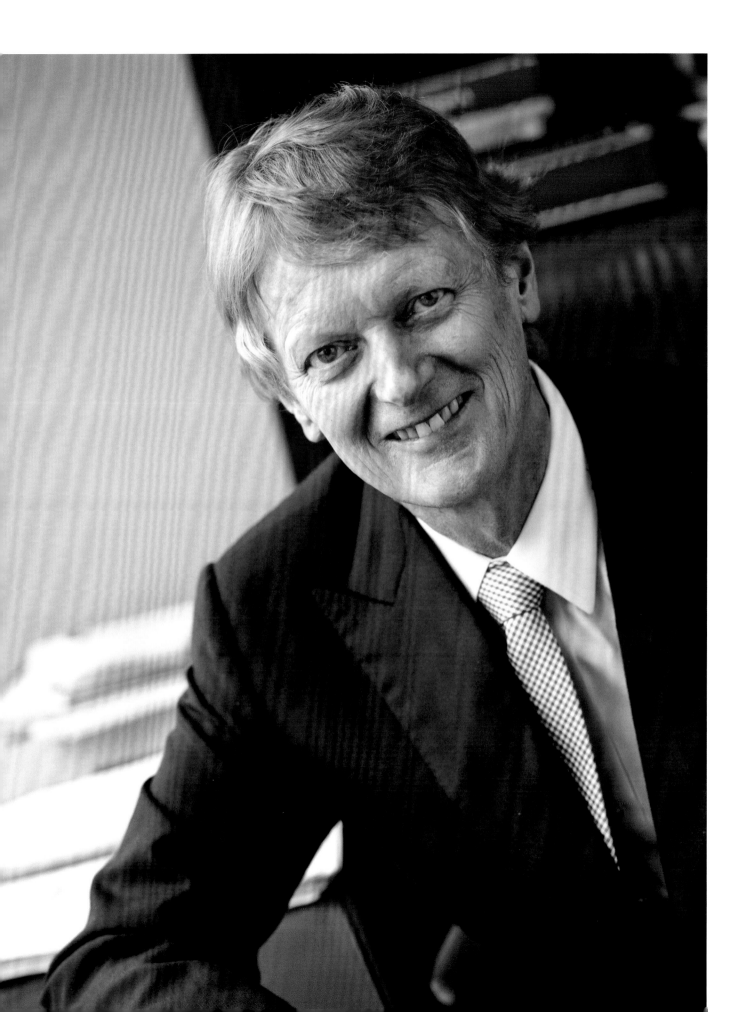

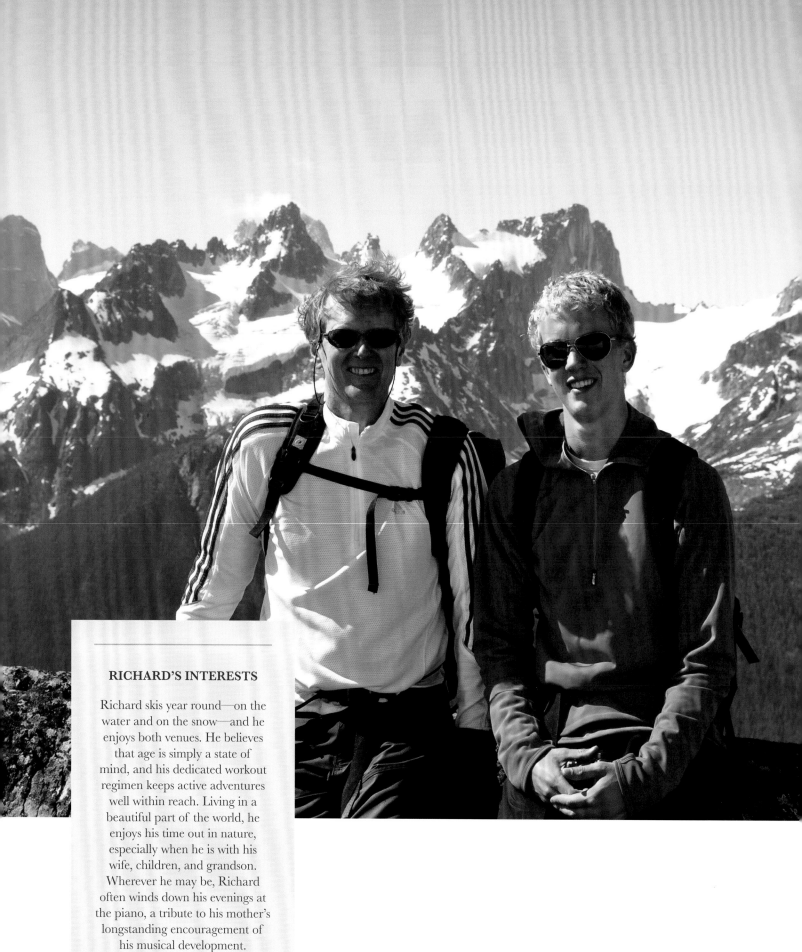

## RICHARD'S INTERESTS

Richard skis year round—on the water and on the snow—and he enjoys both venues. He believes that age is simply a state of mind, and his dedicated workout regimen keeps active adventures well within reach. Living in a beautiful part of the world, he enjoys his time out in nature, especially when he is with his wife, children, and grandson. Wherever he may be, Richard often winds down his evenings at the piano, a tribute to his mother's longstanding encouragement of his musical development.

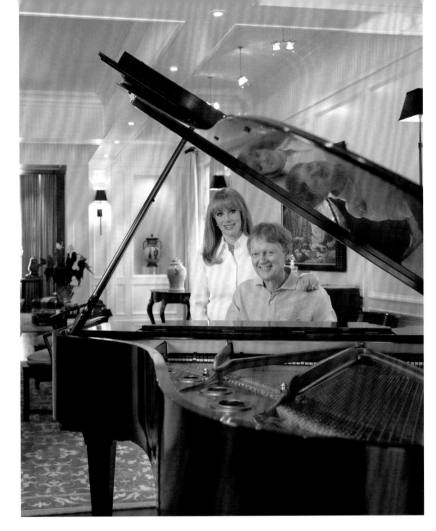

LIKE MANY IN THE industry, Richard is intrigued by historical concepts of beauty and the timelessness of certain principles. However, he also believes that the perception of beauty is highly individual. "Every woman has her own look—wardrobe, hair, makeup, even the way she carries herself—and she has developed that look based on what she thinks makes her attractive," he explains. "What she may or may not realize, or admit, is that society is telling her what to think." Perceptions on beauty have varied widely through the ages. The hearty and voluptuous women so characteristic of a Rubens painting are fascinating when contrasted with the fuller waistlines and smaller breasts of elegant Greek and Roman statuary, each image reflecting the public sentiment of the time. Today, most of the images we see in the media are not only unreal, they are virtually impossible to achieve. "Even the most beautiful people you see in a magazine are photo-edited beyond recognition—after the photographer's flattering lighting setup and the makeup artist's professional application—and many of the results are not obtainable even with surgery," Richard says. He knows his patients live in a society that makes the standard of beauty unreachable, and he is sensitive to their perceptions as well as their dreams.

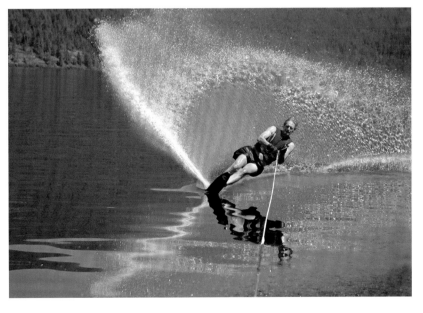

Realistic expectations are of utmost importance to Richard, and merely explaining the potential outcome isn't enough. He shows patients images of results that are average, better than average, and worse than average, offering a candid prediction of what they can expect based on their specific skin or body type. He believes that surgeons should offer patients truthful estimations of what surgery can do now, as well as how the surgical result will evolve over time. For Richard, cosmetic surgery is not as simple as giving patients what they want. Rather, it's a dialogue that considers society's influence, the patient's desires, the surgeon's strategic recommendations, and—most importantly—the patient's physical and emotional well-being.

The magic Richard tries to deliver is to make people look better without any sign that they had plastic surgery, because, as he says, "good plastic surgery is never obvious."

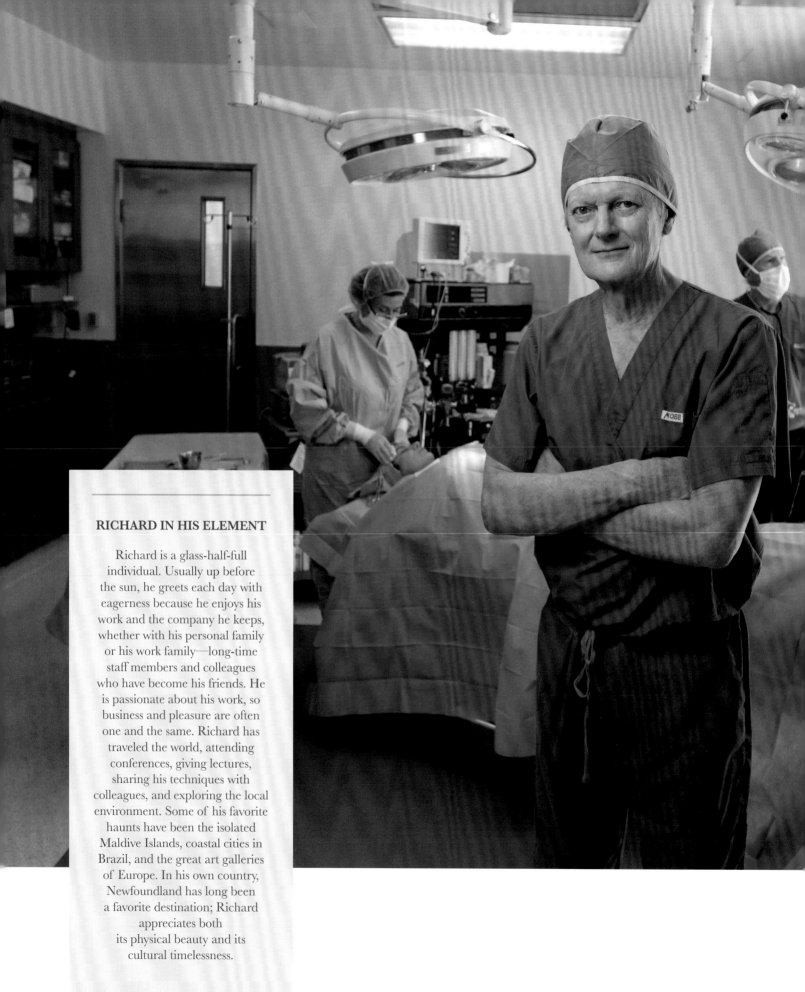

## RICHARD IN HIS ELEMENT

Richard is a glass-half-full individual. Usually up before the sun, he greets each day with eagerness because he enjoys his work and the company he keeps, whether with his personal family or his work family—long-time staff members and colleagues who have become his friends. He is passionate about his work, so business and pleasure are often one and the same. Richard has traveled the world, attending conferences, giving lectures, sharing his techniques with colleagues, and exploring the local environment. Some of his favorite haunts have been the isolated Maldive Islands, coastal cities in Brazil, and the great art galleries of Europe. In his own country, Newfoundland has long been a favorite destination; Richard appreciates both its physical beauty and its cultural timelessness.

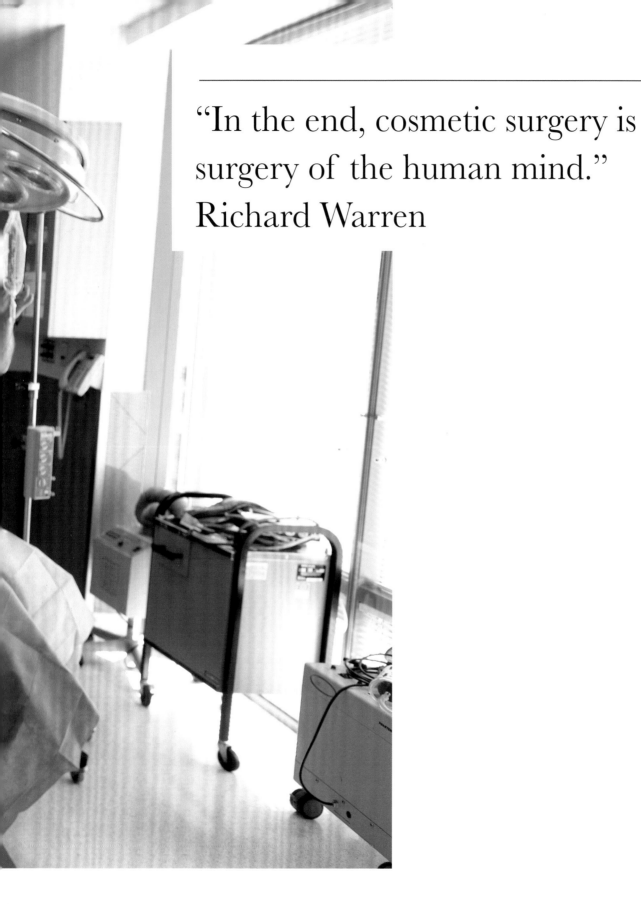

"In the end, cosmetic surgery is surgery of the human mind."
Richard Warren

"Patients will take a very active role in their own well-being and will not look to doctors to 'fix' as many things."
Tracy Pfeifer

# THE DISTANT FUTURE

## WHAT DOES THE INDUSTRY LOOK LIKE IN 50 YEARS?

**Ashley Gordon:** Surgery will be obsolete because we'll be practicing regenerative medicine. The genetics of aging will be fully understood, so everything will be about prevention and not correction. Your robotic plastic surgeon will make house calls in a self-driving car to inject stem cells and growth factors to maintain your "ageless beauty." Men will never go bald, and women won't have cellulite. I hope I live to 100 to witness it.

**Adam Rubinstein:** In 50 years, the science of medicine will offer choices for rejuvenation that don't require a knife or even a syringe. Topical treatments will exist to provide fantastic improvements to the skin: Botox effects without injections, and possibly plumping options without using fillers. We may very well have pills to refresh our appearance in a number of ways to safely rejuvenate without any other intervention at all.

**Clyde Ishii:** More space-age types of noninvasive treatments. Possible gene manipulation to slow down the aging process. Surgery will still have its place in the cosmetic surgery armamentarium.

**Jim Grotting:** Clearly, the trend in the industry is a major surge in nonsurgical procedures that can be done more simply and at less cost than surgery. Unfortunately, those procedures as of this writing cannot deliver the powerful results of surgery. Nevertheless, they are improving, and as skin tightening is able to be done without scars, we will be closer to the "Holy Grail" of aesthetic treatments. We are also recognizing how to improve the health, color, and texture of the skin. These interventions along with timely, well-done surgery can keep a person looking really great throughout life.

**Tracy Pfeifer:** Patients and physicians alike will know more about aging and how to live a healthier lifestyle so that we look and feel better as we age. Patients will take a very active role in their own well-being and will not look to doctors to "fix" as many things. I pray that liposuction and bariatric weight loss surgery is a thing of the past, as everyone maintains a healthy weight on their own through proper nutrition and exercise. There is no reason for liposuction except in very specific times when diet-resistant fat tissue needs to be removed. Similarly, bariatric surgery should never be necessary. It is a byproduct of unhealthy eating habits.

**Sheila Nazarian:** Noninvasive and preventative treatments are really taking over. I can imagine a lot less surgery will be needed in 50 years.

**Richard Warren:** In 50 years, I suspect we won't recognize many of the cosmetic procedures we do today. Some possibilities I can imagine include genetic alterations to extend life, manmade body parts (3D printing using collagen/bone or fat substitutes), synthetic inserts to make facelifts last longer, better breast implants that last forever and never go hard, better methods to remove fat, and improved methods to re-insert fat grafts that will make the results more predictable. I suspect there will be more and better science behind the marketing of cosmeceuticals. The industry will have grown, and there will probably be more and different kinds of doctors supplying the services we now provide. I don't think robotic surgery will have much of a place in cosmetic surgery, so I can imagine that, in 50 years, there will still be a long course of surgical training for plastic surgeons. Perhaps surgical simulation will be more prevalent in surgical training, but in the end, someone is going to have to pick up surgical instruments and do the work themselves. That will always require extensive hands-on training.

**Anna Petropoulos:**
Bioengineering, stem cells, possibly even genomics might start being implemented for beauty. Just recently, a monkey was cloned just like Dolly the Sheep. Be it right or wrong, using genomics for beauty is going way beyond my philosophy of just using no-risk, safe, noninvasive techniques of maintaining what God gave us.

> "In 50 years? No downtime, no pain, amazing results."
> Robyn Siperstein-Paul

## Ashley Gordon, MD, F.A.C.S.

Board Certified Plastic Surgeon
Restora Austin Plastic Surgery Centre
901 W. 38th Street, Suite 401
Austin, Texas 78705
512.371.8817
restoraaustin.com
Instagram: @restoraaustin
Facebook: Restora Austin

## James C. Grotting, MD, F.A.C.S.

Director, The American Board of Plastic Surgery
Past President, The American Society for
Aesthetic Plastic Surgery
Grotting & Cohn Plastic Surgery
1 Inverness Center Parkway
Birmingham, Alabama 35242
205.930.1600
grottingplasticsurgery.com
grottingcohnplasticsurgery.com
Instagram: @jamesgrotting

## Clyde H. Ishii, MD, F.A.C.S.

President, The American Society for Aesthetic Plastic Surgery
CHI Plastic Surgery Center
1329 Lusitana Street, Suite 304
Honolulu, Hawaii 96813
808.537.6630
ishiiplasticsurgery.com

## John Koutsoyiannis, DDS

sohosmile
206 Spring Street, 5th Floor
New York, New York 10012
212.334.7330
www.sohosmile.com

## Charles S. Lee, MD, F.A.C.S.

Enhance Medical Center, Inc.
462 N. Linden Drive, Suite 333
Beverly Hills, California 90212
310.271.5954
enhanceplasticsurgery.com
asiancosmeticsurgery.com
Instagram: @drlee90210

## Sheila Nazarian, MD, MMM

Board Certified Plastic Surgeon
Nazarian Plastic Surgery
120 South Spalding Drive, Suite 315
Beverly Hills, California 90212
310.659.0500
nazarianplasticsurgery.com
theskinspot.com
Instagram: @drsheilanazarian
Facebook: Nazarian Plastic Surgery

## Anna Petropoulos, MD, FRCS

The New English Facial & Cosmetic Surgery Center
80 Lindall Street, Suite 1 & 2
Danvers, Massachusetts 01923
978.739.9500
classicface.com
Instagram: @centerforclassicbeauty

## Tracy Pfeifer, MD, MS

Board Certified Plastic Surgeon
Board Member, The American Society for Aesthetic Plastic
Surgery
Past President, New York Regional Society of Plastic Surgeons
Pfeifer Plastic Surgery
1175 Park Avenue, Suite 1B
New York, New York 10128
212.860.0670
drpfeifer.com
breastsurgeryrevisions.com
Instagram: @drtracypfeifer
Twitter: @DrTracyPfeifer
Facebook: Dr. Tracy Pfeifer

## Marta I. Rendon, MD, FACP, FAAD

President Elect, Women's Dermatological Society
Rendon Center for Dermatology and Aesthetic Medicine
1001 NW 13 Street, Suite 100
Boca Raton, Florida 33486
561.750.0544
drrendon.com
rendoncenter.com
Instagram: @rendoncenter
Facebook: Rendon Center for Dermatology
and Aesthetic Medicine

## Adam J. Rubinstein, MD, F.A.C.S.
2999 NE 191st Street, PH6
Miami, Florida 33180
305.792.7575
dr-rubinstein.com
Instagram: @drrubinstein; @plasticsurgerytruths
Snapchat: @drrubinstein
Facebook: MiamiPlasticSurgeon

## Robyn Siperstein-Paul, MD
Board Certified Dermatologist
Founder, Siperstein Dermatology Group
950 Glades Road, 4th Floor
Boca Raton, Florida 33431
561.955.8885
sipderm.com
Instagram: @sip_derm
Twitter: @SipDermGroup
Facebook: Siperstein Dermatology

## Armando Soto, MD, F.A.C.S.
Director, Aesthetic Enhancements Plastic Surgery
and Skin Care Center
7009 Dr. Phillips Boulevard, Suite 100
Orlando, Florida 32819
407.218.4550
drarmandosoto.com
Instagram: @drsoto_orlando

## Charles H. Thorne, MD
812 Park Avenue
New York, New York 10021
212.794.0044
charlesthornemd.com
microtia.com

## Jennifer L. Walden, MD, F.A.C.S., PLLC
Walden Cosmetic Surgery and Laser Center
5656 Bee Cave Road, Suite E201
Austin, Texas 78746
512.328.4100
drjenniferwalden.com
themedspaaustin.com
Instagram: @drjenniferwalden
Twitter: @drjenwalden
Facebook: Dr. Jennifer Walden

## Richard J. Warren, MD, FRCSC
Clinical Professor of Surgery, University of British Columbia
Past President, Canadian Society for Aesthetic Plastic Surgery
Past Chairman, Canadian Specialty Board for Plastic Surgery
Director, Vancouver Plastic Surgery Center
777 West Broadway, Suite 1000
Vancouver, British Columbia, Canada V5Z4J7
604.876.1774
drrichardjwarren.com
vancouverplasticsurgerycenter.com

"The more one learns and sees and appreciates, the more elusive perfection becomes."

Charles Thorne